# TABLE OF CONTENTS

# INTRODUCTION

Welcome to One Good Turn's Corona Care Handbook. We are so glad to share this wealth of strategies to help you deal with COVID-19. One Good Turn is an international health care organization located in Austin, Texas. Our team provides basic medical education to underserved communities around the world. We work with nurses, school health workers, village leaders, and clinicians. We provide practical and effective medical plans using whatever resources are available in places where even electricity is a luxury. When COVID-19 first emerged, One Good Turn's immediate concern was for our global partners. In the at-risk, neglected communities where we work, there are no hospitals or ventilators, and there are very few doctors. So we began sharing simple, practical methods to help prevent and treat COVID-19 without fancy medications or machines.

Soon, we were fielding urgent questions from friends and associates right here in America: What is this Corona thing? Who can we trust to give us accurate advice? What can we do to protect and treat ourselves? Like you, we watched in shock and astonishment as the virus spread throughout the world. This pandemic is confusing, often frightening, and disruptive to each of us in different ways. COVID-19 is a global health crisis that has no boundaries.

In response, One Good Turn has added "home" to our global health network. We review high-level medical research; write COVID-19 response guidelines for businesses, shelters, and families here in the US; and share new developments and practical tips through the press, social media, and our website. The perceptive questions and enthusiastic responses we've gotten are inspiring. Clearly, people want practical information about how to cope with COVID-19. And so, just as we do with all our projects, we wrote a handbook for our new community partners: YOU, our friends and family here at home.

Inside this Corona Care Handbook, you will find practical action plans designed for the vast majority of people who will handle COVID-19 without ever going to a doctor or hospital or being put on a ventilator. Someday, there will be a vaccine and other effective medical treatments. Right now, we must rely on our ingenuity, the resources we already have, and our concern for one another to prevail over this pandemic.

- Ann Messer, MD
Founder and Executive Director
One Good Turn

# HOW TO USE THIS HANDBOOK:

We've organized this guide book into chapters based on the situations you will encounter as you deal with the pandemic in your daily life. Look through the Table of Contents and turn to whatever chapter you need. Of course, we hope you'll read it all! The information is cross-referenced so that you will always be able to find the right breathing exercise or disinfecting solution, no matter where you are in the book. Really sick? Have to go to work? Need to track your symptoms? You'll find what you need in our handbook.

Because information is developing so rapidly, **the reference links in this handbook are live. Please check them regularly.** The world's knowledge and understanding of this new virus is changing frequently; stay updated by checking reliable sources: the CDC, the WHO, your state's public health department, and One Good Turn. This handbook was published in August of 2020. Compare this date to any new information you find.

Stay calm, stay connected; we are all in this together. One Good Turn is on your team! Contact us with questions or comments - One Good Turn believes in the power of community and information sharing. We value your thoughts and welcome your input.

# WHAT IS COVID-19?

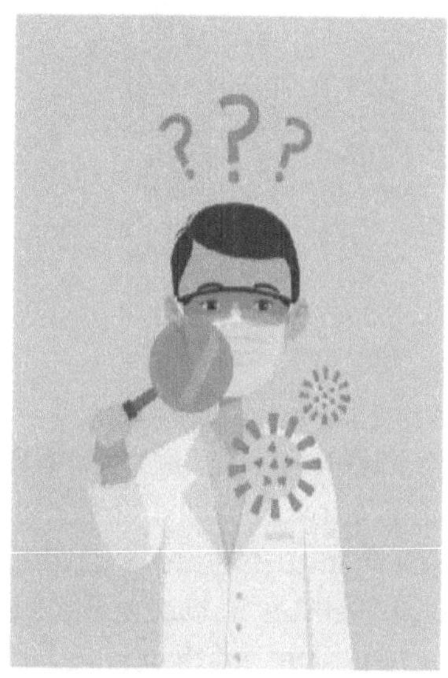

## Chapter 1 Outline

1) What is COVID-19?

2) Virus Replication

3) The Human Body's Response to the Virus

    a) Pneumonia

    b) Cytokine Storm

4) Virus Spread/Transmission

5) Contagious Period and Isolation/Quarantine

## 6) Virus on Surfaces

Understanding how COVID-19 grows, spreads, and infects people can make it easier to protect yourself. First, let's take a look at the COVID-19 virus itself. Then we will go over how the virus grows inside the body (replication) and the basics of the illness it causes. Finally, we'll discuss how COVID-19 spreads (transmission).

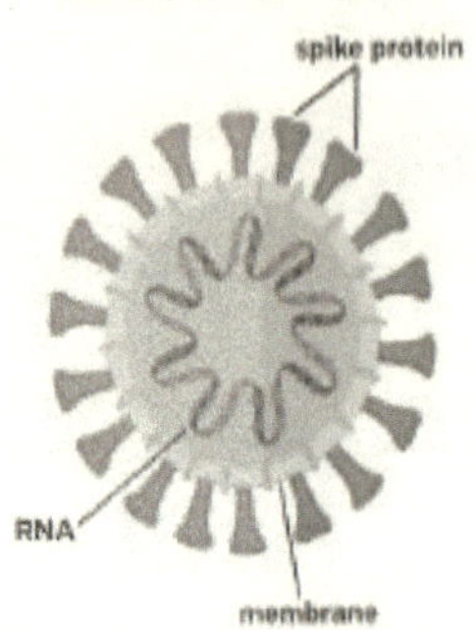



COVID-19 is a new form of coronavirus, the family of germs that causes infections like the common cold, the flu, and some kinds of pneumonia. We've all had a coronavirus or two! Just like the cold and flu viruses, COVID-19 will continue to change (mutate), but the basics of how the virus spreads and infects people will stay the same. Because COVID-19 is a new form of the virus, we humans have not developed any immunity to it - our infection-fighting cells don't yet know how to respond.

A virus is not a living cell. It's a pretty amazing little piece of biologic machinery with the single mission to make copies of itself. The COVID-19 virus has **3 basic parts**: sharp **spikes**, which attach onto living cells; **RNA,** which acts like a computer code trying to hack into and take over the cells it contacts; and a thin **membrane**, which holds everything together as the virus moves from cell to cell.

COVID-19 is dangerous because there are many receptors on human cells (ACE-2 receptors) where the virus can latch on and begin an attack. These COVID-19 receptors are located on cells in the nose, throat, eyes, lungs, intestines, blood vessels, and many other parts of the body.

This makes sense when we think about the symptoms that are commonly seen with COVID-19, which occur in all the places where people have receptors! These receptor cells are also the sites from which the virus spreads out of a sick person's body to other people.

# Virus Replication

The viral replication process goes through four stages (you can see them in the drawing below):

1. **Entry into the human cell** - The spikes on the surface of the COVID virus latch onto a human cell, causing the viral membrane to open ribbon of RNA code to enter the cell.

2. **Takeover of the human cell** - The RNA ribbon takes command of t machinery to make new RNA copies of the virus.

3. **Multiplication of the virus** - These copies multiply into a thousand particles.[1]

4. **Destruction of the human cell** - Swollen with virus particles, the h cell finally bursts open, releasing these new viral particles into the s where they attack other cells inside the body and continue multiply

# HOW COVID-19 REPLICATES INSIDE THE BODY

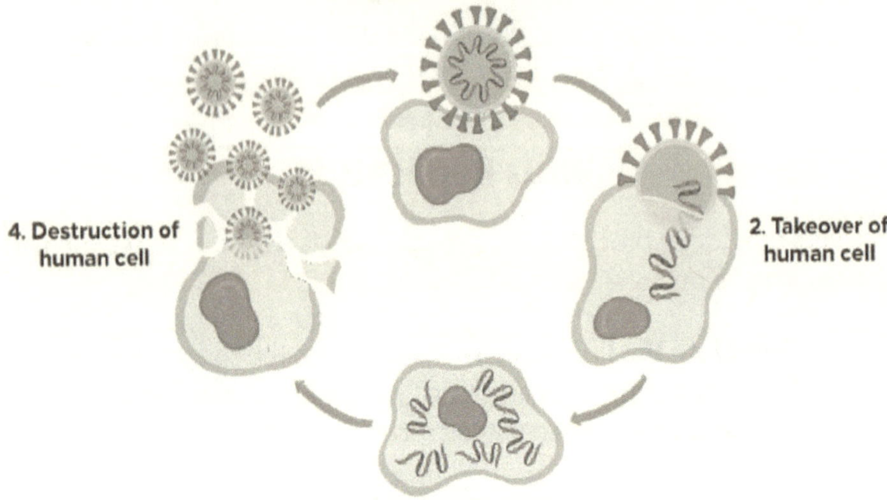



## The Human Body's Response to the Virus

So much cellular debris is created in this replication process - hundreds of thousands of broken cells and millions of viral particles - that the human body's immune response is activated and creates a flood of fighter cells and fluids, which rush to the sites where the virus is attacking. The debris and inflammation cause the basic symptoms of COVID-19: fever, sore throat, loss of taste and smell, cough, diarrhea, and fatigue.

Two responses can cause dangerous - even deadly - complications of COVID-19.

## Pneumonia

COVID-19 loves the lungs. Full of receptor sites for the virus, the warm, dark, air-filled areas at the base of the lungs are a great spot for viral growth (replication). If the virus attacks the lungs, it can cause fluid buildup, inflammation, and serious infection. This attack can happen very suddenly, and the infection can block oxygen exchange in the lungs. People who can't get enough oxygen are rushed to the hospital. They need supplemental oxygen, IV fluids, and sometimes even intubation (where oxygen is delivered to the lungs through a large tube with enough pressure to push past all the fluid and infection). This is called ARDS: Acute Respiratory Distress Syndrome.

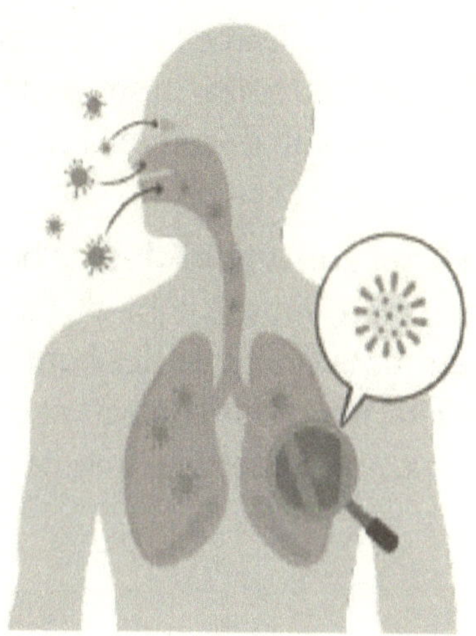

## Cytokine Storm

The human immune system, not sure of what to do to stop this new virus, sends a huge wave of fighter cells and breakdown chemicals to the sites of infection. This creates excessive inflammation all over the body, in important organs like the kidneys, the intestines, the brain, and the blood vessels. The body can't cope. Patients develop fatigue, confusion, muscle pain, high fever, and organ failure (MODS - Multiple Organ Dysfunction Syndrome).

Thankfully, the vast majority of people infected with COVID-19 will not die.

Most people will be able to stay at home to recover. Some folks will have few symptoms, or even none. Recovery will happen in a few weeks, not the months it takes to resolve serious illness. Yet **a person with a mild infection can pass COVID-19 to someone who will end up on a ventilator.** Why is this? Here are the leading theories:

- People with risk factors (older age, illness, etc.) can't fight off the virus as well.

- People with overactive immune systems (allergies, asthma, etc.) have too much of an immune response since their systems are already revved up.

- People whose bodies produce a higher **viral load** (the total number of viral particles that are replicated in the body) have more virus to fight off. Recently published research shows a higher viral load in lung fluids from patients with pneumonia compared to those without pneumonia.

- People who get a higher **infectious dose** (a bigger initial load of virus particles) have more virus to fight off. For example, an individual who gets more virus particles from one very contagious person or from several infectious contacts at once (like in a nursing home, hospital, or close work setting) may have a higher initial infectious dose.

## Virus Spread/Transmission

So, how does COVID-19 spread? Here's a demonstration to try: breathe out of your mouth and onto a mirror or a glass surface. Do you see that steam on the glass? If you have COVID-19, that steam is full of contagious viral particles!

COVID-19 spreads from person to person when the virus leaves an infected person's nose, mouth, and/or lungs. In the air, the moisture and virus particles are called "droplets" (which can be bigger and goopier when someone coughs or sneezes). Once they land on a surface (like your fingers, your phone, or a table), they are called "fomites."

The virus that causes COVID-19 spreads very easily between people. This spread of infection is called the "viral transmission process." It occurs when an infected person passes the virus to other people either directly (when droplets in the air are inhaled by an uninfected person) or indirectly (when fomites on surfaces are touched by an uninfected person who then touches their face/nose/mouth and inhales the infected droplet). It only takes a few viral particles - estimates are as little as 10 and up to 1,000 - to infect someone. This is significant because a person can expel about 30,000 droplets when they sneeze!

## Contagious Period and Isolation/Quarantine

The contagious period is the time that an infected person can spread virus particles to others. For COVID-19, since the virus quickly multiplies inside the body, a "pre-symptomatic" period is thought to begin 2-3 days before the infected person develops symptoms. **It is because of this symptom-free contagious period that wearing face masks, hand-washing, and social distancing are so important.** This symptom-free period is also another reason this illness spreads so quickly!

Scientists believe that the contagious period lasts for about 10 days after symptoms start and even longer if the cough and fever continue. This is the basis for the CDC's recommendation that an infected person stay in **isolation** for **10 days** after symptoms have started or after a positive COVID-19 viral test (see Chapter 3: Test!) even if the person isn't showing symptoms.[2]

The **quarantine** period is the length of time that a person who has possibly been exposed to an infected person must stay away from others.[3] For COVID-19, the quarantine time is **14 days**. Quarantine is longer than isolation because it includes the 2-3 days of pre-symptomatic spread as well as the 10 day illness (regardless of symptoms). People in quarantine should stay home, separate themselves from others, monitor their health, and follow directions from their state or local health department.

## Virus on Surfaces

Droplets and fomites are contagious until the fragile viral membranes are broken down by soap, hand sanitizer, disinfectant, heat, sunlight, or time. It may be possible for a person to get COVID-19 by **touching a surface or**

**object that has the virus on it** and then touching their own mouth, nose, or possibly their eyes. This is not thought to be the main way the virus spreads, but we are still learning more about this. That is why routinely cleaning and disinfecting frequently touched surfaces is recommended by the CDC.[4] See <u>Chapter 2</u>: Yikes! for further information.

That's a lot of science, but this basic information lays the foundation for a great COVID-19 response plan. Masks, cleaning solutions, exercises, social distancing, and more - all the details you need are in the following chapters, organized by common situations. Let's explore how to say safe in our challenging new environment.

# YIKES! COVID-19 IS EVERYWHERE

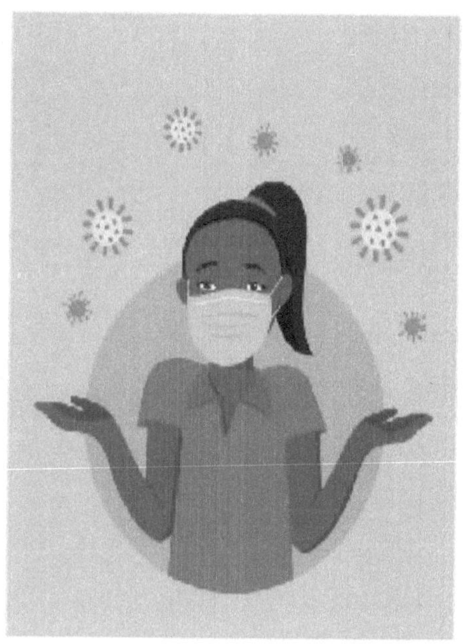

## Chapter 2 Outline

1) All About Personal Protective Equipment
   a) Masks
   b) Glasses/Eye Protection
   c) Gloves
2) Hand Washing

3) Hand Sanitizer

4) Your Environment

    a) COVID-19 and Sunlight

    b) COVID-19 and Sound Volume

    c) At Home

5) Cleaning

    a) Supplies

    b) Cell phones/Electronics

    c) Bathrooms

6) Contact With Others: Social Distancing

    a) Family and Friends

    b) Shopping/Dining

    c) Transportation

    d) Hotels/Travel

    e) Act as if everyone has COVID-19

7) Individuals at Higher Risk

    a) Asthma

    b) Smoking/Vaping

    c) Obesity

    d) Pregnancy

    e) Babies

    f) Maintain your Health

8) Other Ways to Protect Yourself

    a) Make a Daily Prep Kit

    b) Make an Illness Prep Kit

    c) Take your Vitals Now

    d) Supplements

    e) Breathing Exercises

9) Mental Health

    a) Mental Health in Adults

    b) Mental Health in Children

We get it. COVID-19 is scary. With so much new information and more people sick everyday, it's hard to know what to do about COVID-19. This pandemic will affect all of us in many different ways. Knowledge is power, and having a practical response plan will help you keep your home and family safe. Our goal is to help you feel prepared to handle all things COVID-19. Keep this plan close by and share it with others.

The best ways to avoid COVID-19 are pretty simple: Use personal protective equipment, like masks; keep your hands and surfaces around you clean; and control your environment by limiting contact with others outside of your socially distanced bubble. **Simple, but not easy!**

# All About Personal Protective Equipment

## Masks

Our nose has 2 sets of cells inside it - goblet and ciliated cells - that are key entry points for the COVID-19 virus. COVID-19 attaches right onto those cells and then multiplies exponentially and travels down into the lungs. This is why it is so important for your mask to cover your mouth AND your nose!

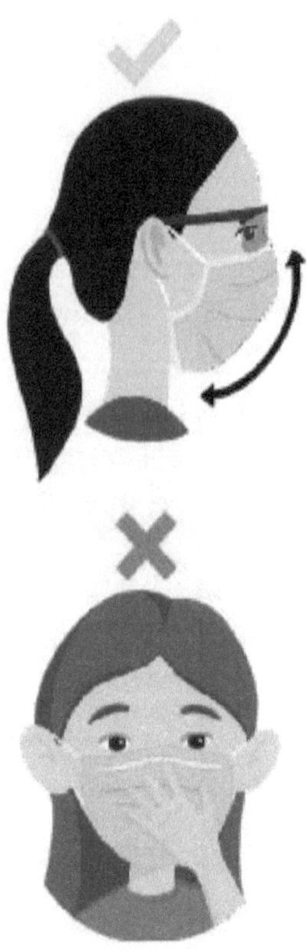

If you leave your nose outside of your mask, you're exposing these key entry points to the COVID-19 virus, which means you're putting yourself at risk of infection. Make sure your mask fits tightly under your chin and OVER your nose without gaps on the side of your face.

Don't touch the front of your mask - that's where COVID-19 virus collects instead of infecting you!

Another benefit of the mask is that it can help you form the habit of **NOT touching your face** - an important habit to minimize viral exposure. Did you know that on average, people touch their faces 18 times an hour? That's once every 3 minutes! This is a difficult habit to change, but now that you know about it, it will be easier. Try to avoid touching your face as much as possible, even when wearing a mask. This decreases the chances of inhaling germs or rubbing them into your eyes, nose, or mouth. In addition to using a mask, gloves and scented hand sanitizer or soap can help you remember where your hands are and to keep them away from your face.

## Why are masks so important?

Droplets from an uncovered cough can travel at least 8-12 feet at 50 miles per hour. Sneeze droplets can travel 100 miles an hour! To best protect yourself and others, wear a mask and encourage anyone around you to wear a mask. Even with a mask, cover your coughs or sneezes with your bent elbow. And keep your 6-foot distance - masks don't replace social distancing.

Hospital studies show that when only patients OR health care workers wear masks, there is a high rate of COVID-19 transmission to everyone. However, when everyone - all patients AND all healthcare workers - wear masks, the spread of COVID-19 greatly decreases.[5] This means that COVID-19 transmission is prevented most effectively when **everyone** is wearing a mask.[6]

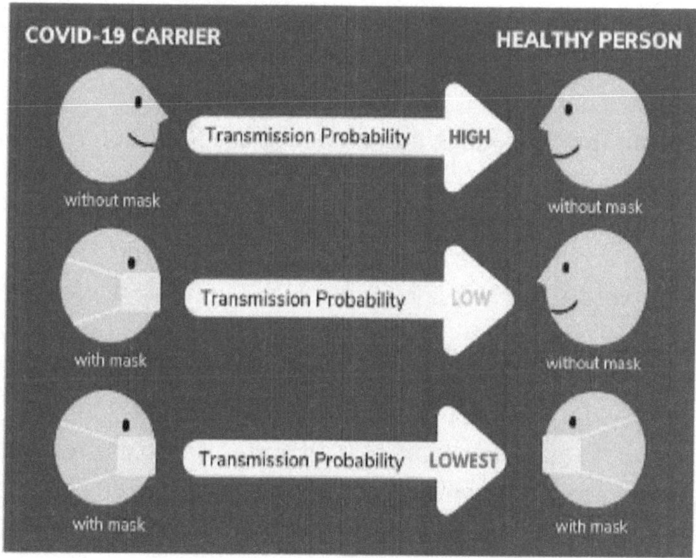


**Tip:** If you accidentally come into close contact with another person or realize someone is near you without a mask on, hold your breath without inhaling. After moving 6 feet away, start to breathe again by exhaling first.

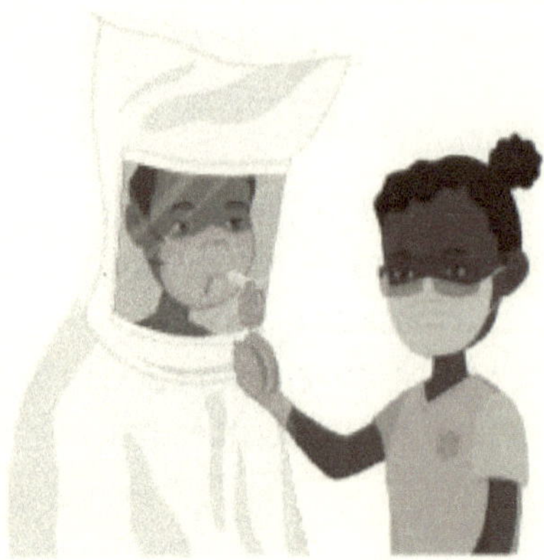

## Types of Masks

* **N95**: These masks are specific for healthcare providers' use in the hospital. These masks only work if they are fit tightly to your face. Do NOT reuse a N95 mask if it gets wet. The filter won't work anymore. NOTE - N95 masks require a special "fit test" to be sized and shaped correctly. This is done for healthcare workers at hospitals - without a fit test you won't know if your N95 is protecting you!

* **Surgical/Medical**: These masks are disposable, looser fitting than N95 masks, and have a special filter. The darker (often blue- or yellow-tinted) side faces outwards and the white side goes against the face. Do NOT reuse a surgical mask if it gets wet; the filter won't work anymore. The outside of the mask should be water resistant, but if you think your mask might have gotten wet, play it safe and get another one. Make sure the mask is big enough to fully cover your lower face. NOTE - There are now lots of these types of masks available in stores. Be aware that **although some masks look like surgical masks, they may not have hospital-grade filters or be water resistant**. Make sure that whatever mask you buy has 3 layers.

* **Cloth**: These masks are made of a variety of materials with a wide range of filtration capabilities. Therefore, cloth masks should have a

filter made of a non-woven fabric sandwiched between 2 layers of cloth. Check that the ear loops are comfortable and will maintain their stretch.

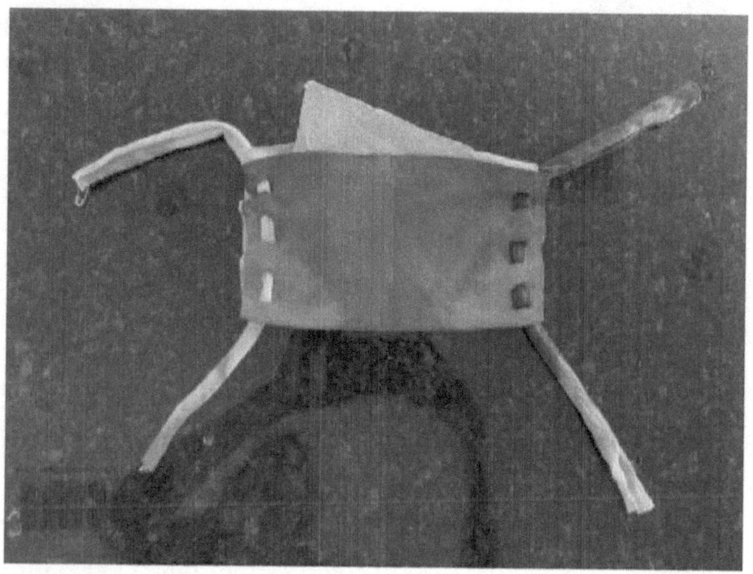

## Instructions for a Basic Cloth Mask

1. Cut a piece of cloth from the fabric choices above that is 2 handspa and 1 wide.

2. Fold it in half (it should fit well under your chin and above your nos

3. Fold each edge and cut 6 small slits on each side.

4. Attach a safety pin or paper clip to one end of the tie.

5. Thread the tie through the slits, like you are lacing up a shoe.

6. Add a filter, such as a paper towel or dish towel (a "non-woven fabr best), to the pocket created by folding the cloth in half as noted in :

7. Pull the ties tightly and tie them behind your head or around your e

8. Make sure there is a tight fit around your nose and under your chin.

9. Add a nosepiece for improved mask fit and comfort. A pipe cleaner flexible paper covered metal strip (often called a <u>tin tie</u>) used for res the top of a bag of coffee or cookies has been found to be effective molding to the shape of your nose. Sew the nosepiece onto the top mask with a few stitches.

**Fabrics to use for cloth masks:**[7]
- Use a fabric that is dense enough to capture viral particles, but breathable enough that you will wear it.
- Perform a "light test" on the fabric to help you decide whether a fabric is a good candidate for a mask. Hold it up to a bright light - if you can see the light through the fibers, it's not a good fabric. If minimal light passes through, like with denim, then the cloth is a tight enough weave to make an effective mask.
- Some highly recommended fabrics that have been tested for mask use include: quilter's cotton, canvas, denim, 600 thread count sheets, and t-shirts (must use 4 layers of t-shirt fabric).
- **Do not use synthetics like nylon, rayon, or polyester** - the fabric threads are too smooth to catch particles.
- Studies have shown that buffs, bandanas, and scarves are the worst alternatives.[8] Droplets from a cough behind a bandana can still travel at least 3 feet. Scarf fabric is woven too loosely and doesn't block virus particles or droplets.

**Filters to use for cloth masks:**
- Choose a filter made from a non-woven material.
- Make sure you can breathe through it, as some filters are harder to breathe through than others and shouldn't be used. Coffee filters are popular, but it takes 3 of them to make a good filter.
- Some highly recommended filters are microfiber towels and blue paper shop towels.
-

Do not reuse paper filters, as they are not washable and easily become damp and ineffective around moisture.

## Mask Precautions

**Do NOT use a mask with a valve** (shown to the right) as you could expel potentially infected air and droplets into your surroundings.

**Cloth face coverings should NOT be placed** on children under the age of 2, anyone who has trouble breathing, or anyone who is unconscious, incapacitated, or otherwise unable to remove their mask without assistance.

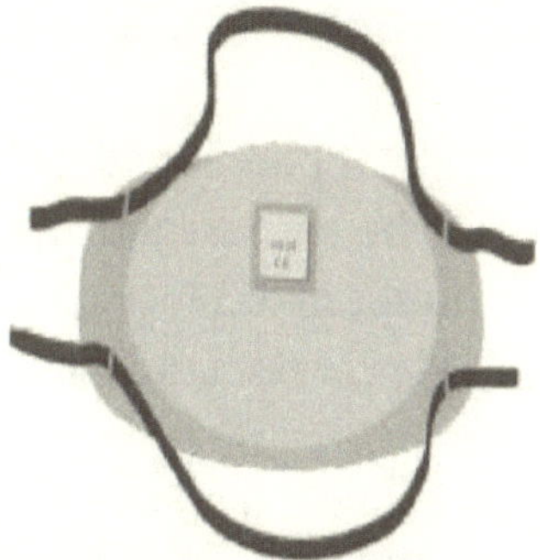

People with **respiratory issues should only use surgical or cloth masks**, as N95 masks are thicker and may cause them to have trouble breathing (N95 masks should be reserved for health workers on the frontline anyway).

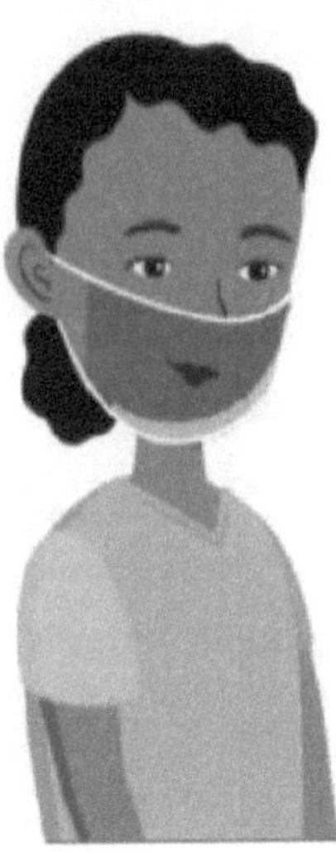

Wearing masks may be difficult for people with sensory, cognitive, or behavioral issues. They should be encouraged to wear a mask, but not forced. Use of face shields and social distancing compliance can help to lessen exposure risks. The CDC now has guidance for this population.[9]

People who are deaf or hard of hearing—or those who care for or interact with a person who is hearing impaired—may be unable to wear masks if they rely on lipreading to communicate. In this situation, consider using a clear mask.[10] If a clear mask isn't available, consider whether you can decrease background noise or use written communication or closed captioning to make communication possible while wearing a mask that blocks your lips.[11]

NOTE - Wearing a face mask should NOT impact your ability to breathe and will not cause carbon dioxide overload.[12,13] Surgical and cloth masks are porous, so air can pass through while droplets carrying virus particles are filtered out. Medical staff all over the world have worn both surgical and N95 masks for hours daily, long before this pandemic. If it feels hard to breathe, step more than 6 feet away from others and adjust your mask. You may interpret the sensation of being able to feel your breath as difficulty breathing. If you need reassurance, check your oxygen saturation before and several minutes after putting on your mask, or when you feel your breathing is uncomfortable. (See <u>Chapter 4</u>: Oh No! for more information on oxygen monitors.) If your oxygen saturation is low, you might need a COVID-19 test. If your oxygen saturation is fine and you still feel uncomfortable, try to adjust your mask - and your attitude - and remind yourself that breathing through a mask is much easier than breathing on a ventilator!

## Normalizing Mask Usage

Masks can feel weird or socially awkward, yet in many parts of the world, protective face coverings are a normal part of life. Here are some tips to help you make the transition. First, make a resolution to protect yourself with a mask (this will increase your success rate by 10 times!). Then, "anchor" your new habit by attaching it to a behavior that's already automatic, like keeping your mask with your chapstick or car keys or putting it on before you open your door. Last, know that repetition is on your side - the more times wear your mask, the faster it will feel normal to you. Get creative! Make a style statement. Finding ways to make wearing a mask fun and interesting will help you to accept this new and important personal accessory.


Tips for adjusting to wearing a mask:

- Be kind to yourself as your body adjusts to wearing a cloth face covering.
- Think positively! Breathing through a mask will feel strange at first. Try to embrace an "I'm going to make this work" mindset.
- Practice wearing a mask at home while watching TV, then try wearing it around the house. Work your way up to taking walks around your neighborhood with your cloth mask. Then try a conversation with a friend. At a store or in public, you may feel nervous at first, and your anxiety might already be high due to fear of exposure. Hang in there!

## Comfort and Fit:

If your current face covering isn't comfortable for you, explore other options. Masks are most comfortable if the area around the nose is well-shaped to your face. The mask needs to fit from the top (bridge) of your nose to all the way under your chin.

**Tip:** Blow out when you put your mask on your face and feel for the places your breath escapes. Tighten those parts up. You can use bobby pins, hair clips, or special straps if you need to pull the loops away from your ears. Shorten the length of ear loops by tying knots to keep the mask close to your face.

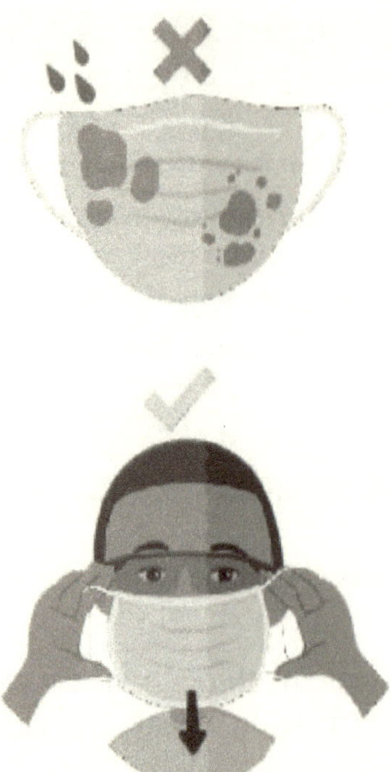

Do not slide the mask up and down on your face - **adjust your mask by pulling up on the ear loops if it does that annoying slip-down-the-nose slide.** Also, it may help to tie back long hair so the mask will fit around your ears better. Germs on masks can easily get caught and carried by long hair. Long beards can also make masks fit poorly.

**Effective Mask Use:**[14]

Make sure your mask is secure before putting on gloves and don't touch the front of your mask, as that is where COVID-19 can collect. Change your mask if it gets wet or dirty.

Remove your mask by grabbing the ties/ear loops - never the front - and pulling it away from your face. Wash your hands for at least 20 seconds before putting your mask on and after removing it. Have 4 cloth masks if possible. More is better, so you can always have a clean one handy. Alternate masks so you have clean ones every day; you can keep the others at home in a paper bag for 4 days (the time it takes COVID-19 to deactivate).

**How to take care of your cloth masks:**

Leave your mask in the sun (on the dash of your car, for example) between uses. Direct sunlight breaks down COVID-19 on surfaces; the time this takes varies depending on the surface and the intensity of sunlight. Even 5-30 minutes helps! Regularly wash your masks with laundry soap and water in the washer. Dry them in the dryer or the sun.

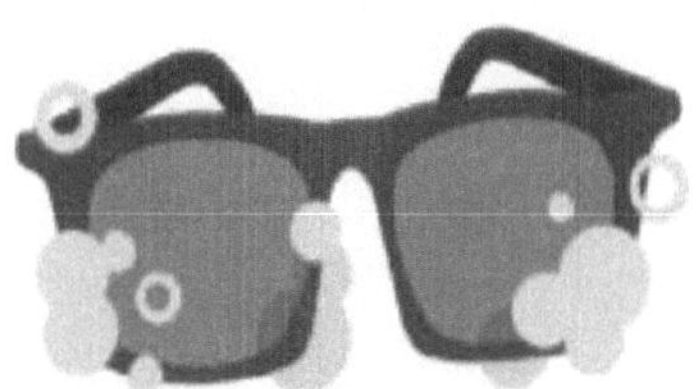

# Glasses/Eye Protection

COVID-19 transmission can happen through the eyes. Goggles are now required for health care workers in many hospitals. Don't touch your eyes and consider using your own glasses, protective shop glasses, or goggles along with your mask when out in public. Face shields also offer great eye and splatter protection, but they do not replace masks - you must wear both. Remember to wash your glasses/face shields regularly with soap or mild alcohol-based cleansers. Be aware that adjusting glasses is a big face-touching risk.

**How to avoid foggy glasses when wearing a mask:**

* Wash glasses with soapy water and let them air dry without rinsing (this works, we tried it!).
* Fold a tissue and place it on the bridge of your nose, underneath your glasses.
* Use a wipe with ethyl alcohol (the ingredient in hand sanitizer) and let the lenses dry fully before putting your glasses on.

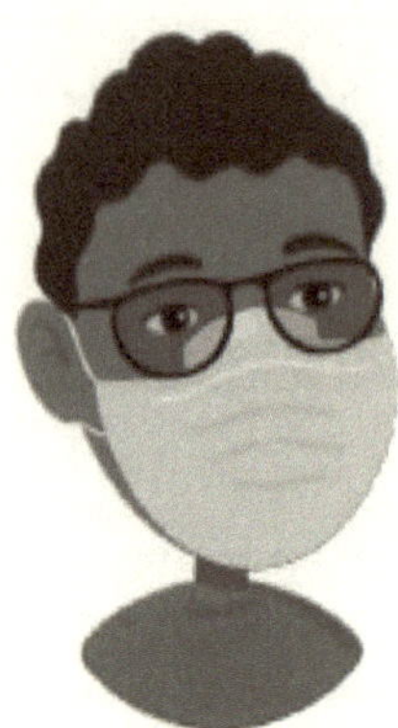

## Gloves

Wearing gloves adds a protective layer between you and surfaces that may carry COVID-19. The trick is to not touch your face or your own things with contaminated gloves. Try wearing 1 glove to touch public surfaces. You can use hand sanitizer on your gloved hands. Rubber or plastic medical-style gloves should only be used once, as they can break down and tear with overuse, washing, and exposure to disinfectant products. Cloth gloves are an excellent option as they are washable, reusable, much more comfortable, and just as protective. Heavier kitchen gloves are great, too. Taking off gloves safely can be tricky; follow this diagram and wash your hands after you toss your glove ball into the trash.

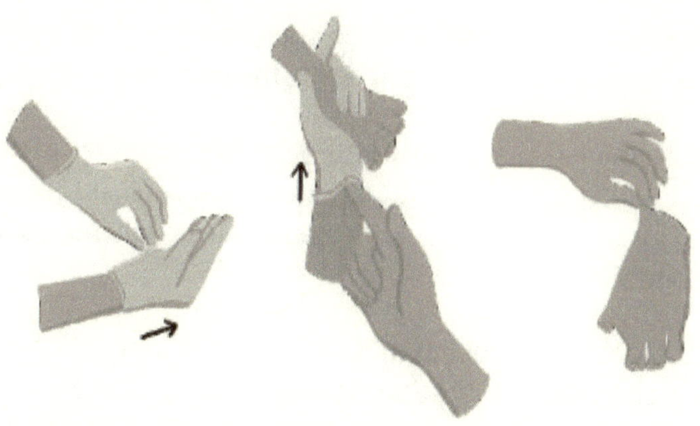

**Tip:** If you are holding a contaminated object (such as a tissue), keep it loosely in your fist as you peel off your glove; it will end up inside your inside-out glove.

## Hand Washing

Washing your hands is one of the best ways to prevent yourself from getting sick and to prevent the spreading of germs to others!

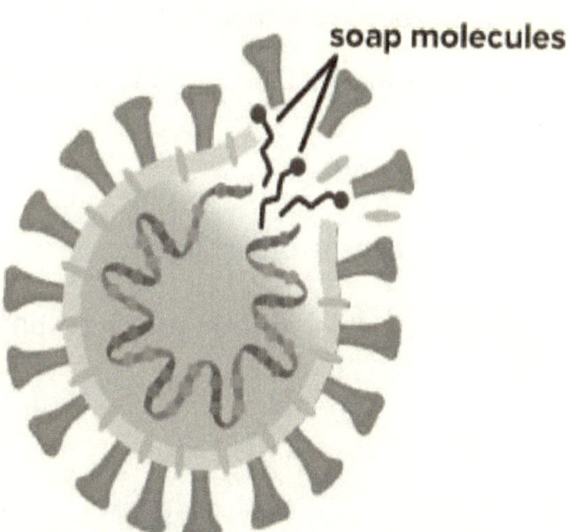


Wash your hands with soap and water whenever possible. **The goal of washing your hands is to use the soap to break down the walls of the**

**COVID-19 virus.** Soap wedges into the outer lipid membrane of the virus. When these membranes are broken down, the virus dies.

Always wash your hands with soap and water when they're visibly dirty, before eating, after using the restroom, after coughing, and before and after caring for anyone who is sick. (Remember to cough into your elbow, not your hands.)

It takes 20 seconds of scrubbing with soap to break down virus walls. **These song choruses are 20 seconds long**: "Take On Me" by A Ha, "Jolene" by Dolly Parton, "Stayin' Alive" by the Bee Gees, "Escape" (The Pina Colada Song) by Rupert Holmes, "Africa" by Toto, "Baby One More Time" by Britney Spears, and "Shake It Off" by Taylor Swift.

And you can never go wrong with Disney songs![15]

**Best Practices for Hand Washing:** (Click here for a link to the CDC video[16])

1. Use enough soap to create a lather with bubbles that covers all par both hands up to above your wrist bone.

2. Rub your hands palm to palm, then one hand over the other.

3. Remember your thumbs!

4. Make sure to scrub between your fingers.

5. Clasp your fingers together to clean your fingertips and under the fingernails.

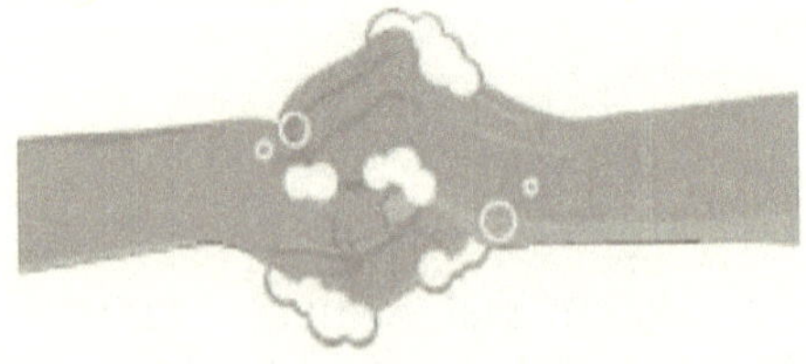

6.  Always scrub for at least 20 seconds. (Save water by turning the wa
    until you're ready to rinse!)

7.  Use a single-use towel to turn the faucet off after washing - you car
    to open the restroom door, too.

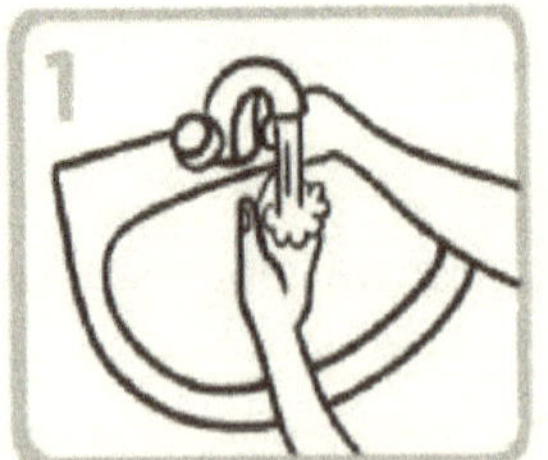

Wet hands with water

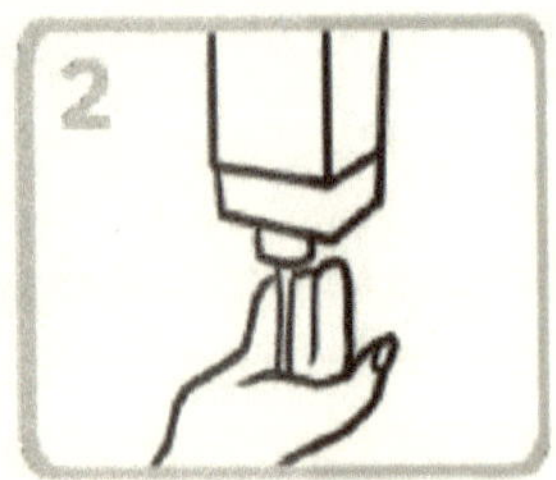

Apply enough soap to cover all hand surfaces

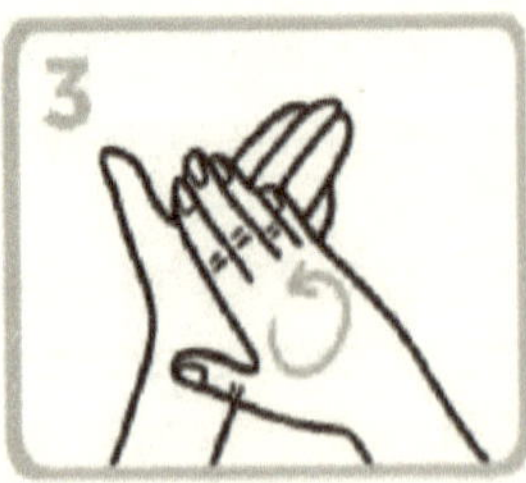

Rub hands palm to palm

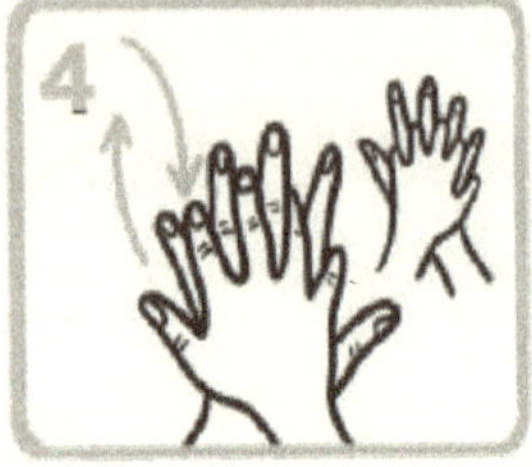

Right palm over left dorsum with interlaced fingers and vice versa

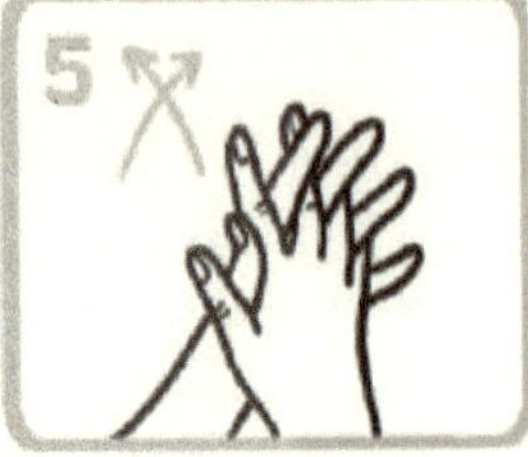

Palm to palm with fingers interlaced

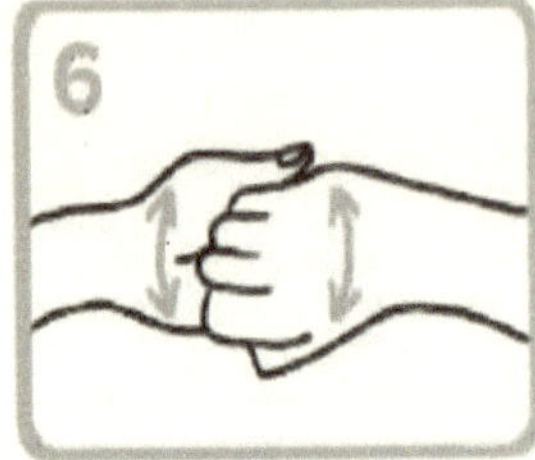

Backs of fingers to opposing palms with fingers interlocked

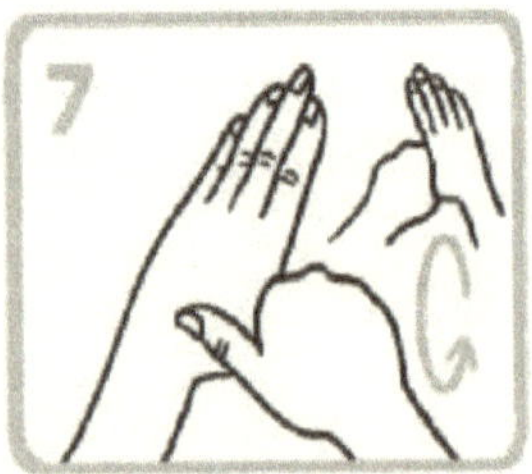

Rotational rubbing of left thumb clasped in right palm and vice versa

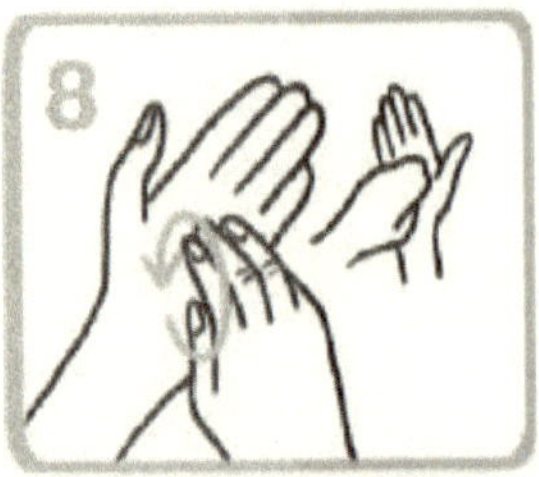

Rotational rubbing, backwards and forwards with clasped fingers of right hand in left palm and vice versa

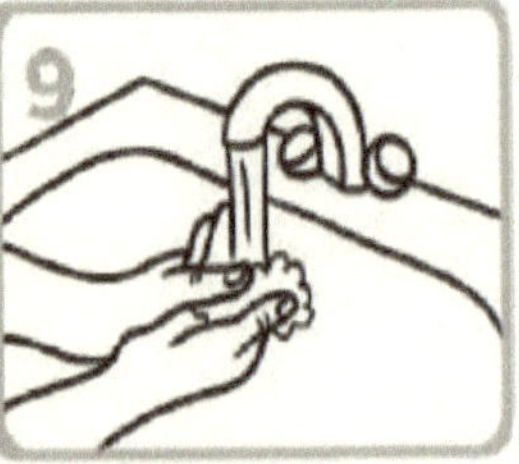

Rinse hands with water

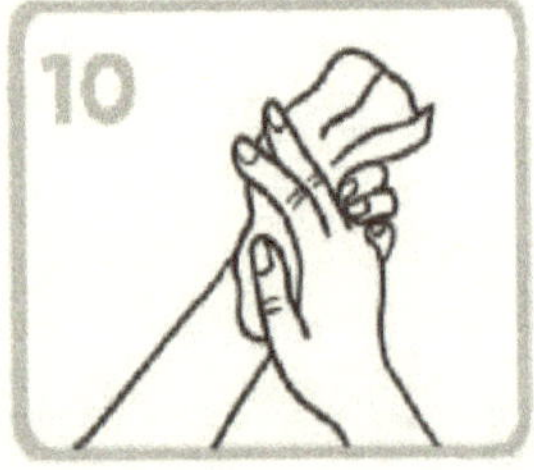

Dry thoroughly with a single towel

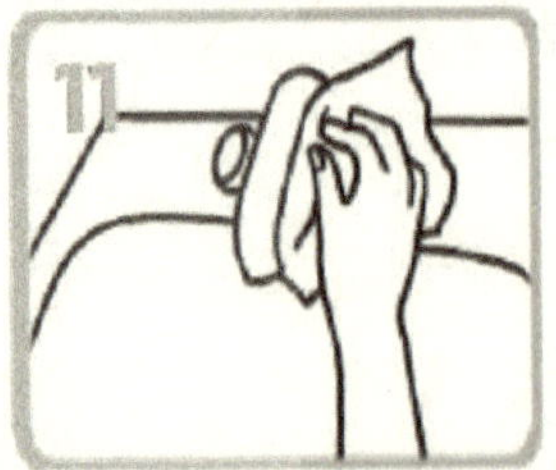

Use towel to turn off faucet

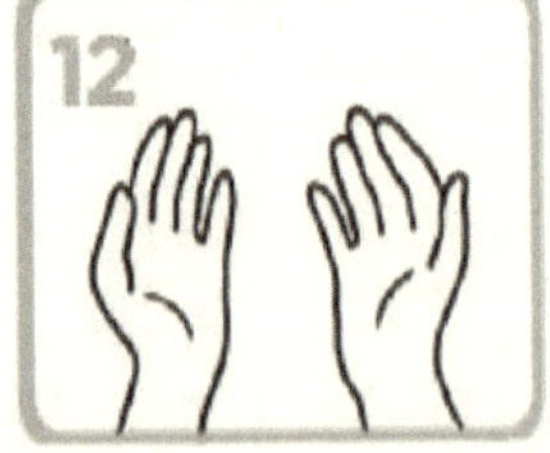

...and your hands are safe.

Buy good-smelling soap for a more pleasant hand washing experience. Fun soaps can turn hand washing into a more entertaining activity, especially if you're trying to teach kids to wash their hands for 20 seconds!

**Tip**: Bar soap works just as well as liquid soap and is MUCH cheaper! Cut up a few bars and carry small pieces if you'll be near a sink during your day.

Soap and water are more effective than hand sanitizers.

# Hand Sanitizer

When soap and water aren't available, use a hand sanitizer with at least 60% alcohol. **The alcohol in hand sanitizer dries out the virus membrane if used effectively.** Alcohol-based hand sanitizers can quickly reduce the number of germs on hands, but sanitizers do not eliminate all germs. Look on the back of the bottle, you'll see the active ingredient "ethyl alcohol," often 60-70%. Less than 60% won't work. Buy a big bottle and a few small travel sized bottles that you can refill.

**Best Practices for Hand Sanitizing:**

- Use enough sanitizer to cover all surfaces of both hands up to the wrist bone.
- Rub between fingers, thumbs, and around fingernails. Use the same technique as for hand washing.
- Allow the sanitizer to dry completely (don't wipe it off!).
- Rub your hands together for at least 20 seconds (or until all sanitizer has dried) to increase friction and kill the maximum amount of active virus.

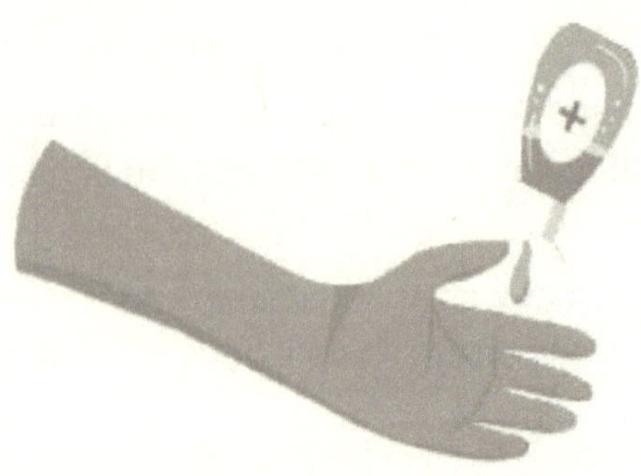

**Warning**: While hand sanitizer can safely have ethanol, some sellers have released hand sanitizers with **methanol, a toxic substance**. Read the FDA list[18] of methanol-containing hand sanitizers - don't buy them! Click here[19] to learn how to make your own hand sanitizer.

**Tip**: If you are without a mask and think you may have just been exposed to COVID-19 (for example, if you are coughed on while in public or a loud group passes close by you in a hallway), put hand sanitizer around your mouth and nose. Dab it on and leave it to dry. Hand sanitizer can be toxic when consumed, so make sure you don't get it in your nose or mouth.

# Your Environment

## COVID-19 and Sunlight

There is much less transmission of COVID-19 in outdoor daytime environments. Direct **sunlight reduces infectious virus particles** after just 3-15 minutes and can destroy COVID-19 droplets on solid surfaces within 30 minutes to 2 hours.[20] If you must have contact with people outside your bubble, try to remain outside in sunlight while practicing social distancing and wearing a mask.

## COVID-19 and Sound Volume

Pay attention to the volume of voices around you! COVID-19 is more likely to be spread through the force of exclamations, singing, and loud voices (especially without masks) because droplets travel farther. Most COVID-19 particles hit the ground by 6 feet away, but studies show that they can remain floating in droplets for up to 18 feet.[21],[22]

## At Home

If you must work and interact with others outside your home, consider keeping a jacket to wear only while you are in high-risk areas like public transportation or crowded markets. Remove and bag it before you enter your home.

When you get home:

* Take off your shoes outside the door.
* Remove potentially exposed clothing and put it in a laundry bag.
* Wash your hands and face - maybe even head to the shower.
* Keep comfortable clothing and slippers to wear only at home.
* If others live in your home and work or interact with others outside the home, ask them to follow these same steps.

It is safe to wash and dry exposed clothing in a machine. Close the laundry bag after adding items. Be sure to wear a mask while doing laundry!

## Cleaning

## Supplies

Wipe down high-use areas regularly with disinfecting wipes or sprays. You can make your own disinfecting solution using household bleach with a sodium hypochlorite concentration of 5%-6%, which is effective against coronaviruses.[23] Dilution is required for safe, appropriate use:

| 5% Liquid Bleach (this is most household bleaches) | Water (at room temperature) |
| --- | --- |

| 1 teaspoon | 1 cup |
| 4 teaspoons | 1 quart |
| ⅓ cup | 1 gallon |

Once you make the bleach solution, it will be effective for disinfection for up to 24 hours. Make a new batch daily as you need it. Some EPA-approved COVID-19 disinfectants include: Scrubbing Bubbles® Multi-Purpose Disinfectant, Fantastik® All-Purpose Cleaner, and Clorox Bleach (click here for more[24]).

**Use thick kitchen gloves with long cuffs** while making or using any disinfectant - bleach is rough on skin. Try protective glasses as well, as bleach fumes can sting your eyes. Keep your cleaning area well ventilated while you work.

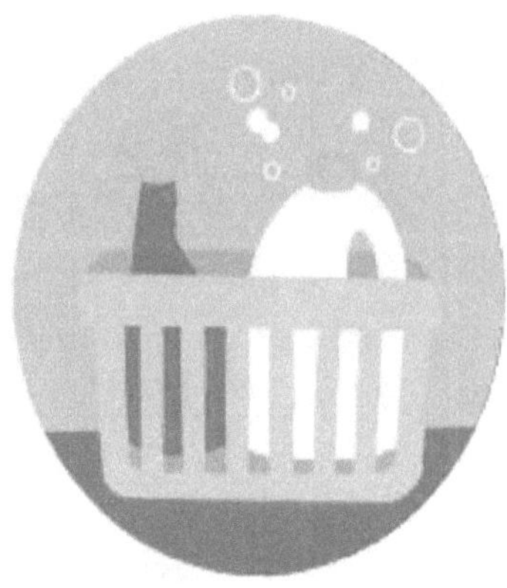

**NOTE - Don't use "low-splash" bleach.** The thickeners make it ineffective against COVID-19.[25,26]

**Look out for fake or ineffective products**! The FDA has a picture list[27] of products that don't work against COVID-19.

It's important to **let your disinfectant sit for 1-5 minutes** to give it time to break down the outer wall of the COVID-19 virus and kill the maximum amount of active virus.[28] Always follow the directions on the label for safety information and application instructions. Keep disinfectants out of the reach of children.

Focus on frequently touched surfaces (such as doorknobs, light switches, lamps, countertops, toilets, and faucets). Clean visibly dirty surfaces with soap and water before disinfecting them. Dishes can be washed in a dishwasher or by gloved hands with hot, soapy water. Areas that are unoccupied for 7 or more days only need routine cleaning. Outdoor areas should continue to be cleaned routinely.

## Cell Phones/Electronics

Try to clean your cell phone every day - it's covered with all kinds of germs and can definitely get contaminated with COVID-19. Many manufacturers have okayed the use of soft 70% alcohol wipes or clorox disinfecting wipes to clean touch screens. Clean any other frequently used electronic devices often as well, especially computer keyboards!

## Bathrooms

Disinfect any surfaces touched after each use. COVID-19 is found in feces, so when toilets are flushed, particles spray into the air. (This is sometimes called a toilet plume!) To protect yourself from these particles, put a long-acting bleach tablet into the toilet tank and close the toilet lid before flushing to minimize spray from the toilet bowl.

## Contact with Others: Social Distancing

The virus that causes COVID-19 spreads very easily between people. In general, the more closely a person interacts with others and the longer that interaction is, the higher the risk of COVID-19 spread.

## Family and Friends

COVID-19 spreads mainly among people who are in close contact (within about 6 feet) for a prolonged period. **Limiting the amount of direct contact with anyone outside of your social distancing bubble to less**

**than 15 minutes is the best way to reduce the spread of COVID-19.**
Remember that if you spend more than 15 minutes within 6 feet of
someone who tested positive for COVID-19, you are a contact and will
need to quarantine for 14 days. Agree with the people in your bubble to
hold each other accountable. Be proud if your gang stays COVID-19
negative!

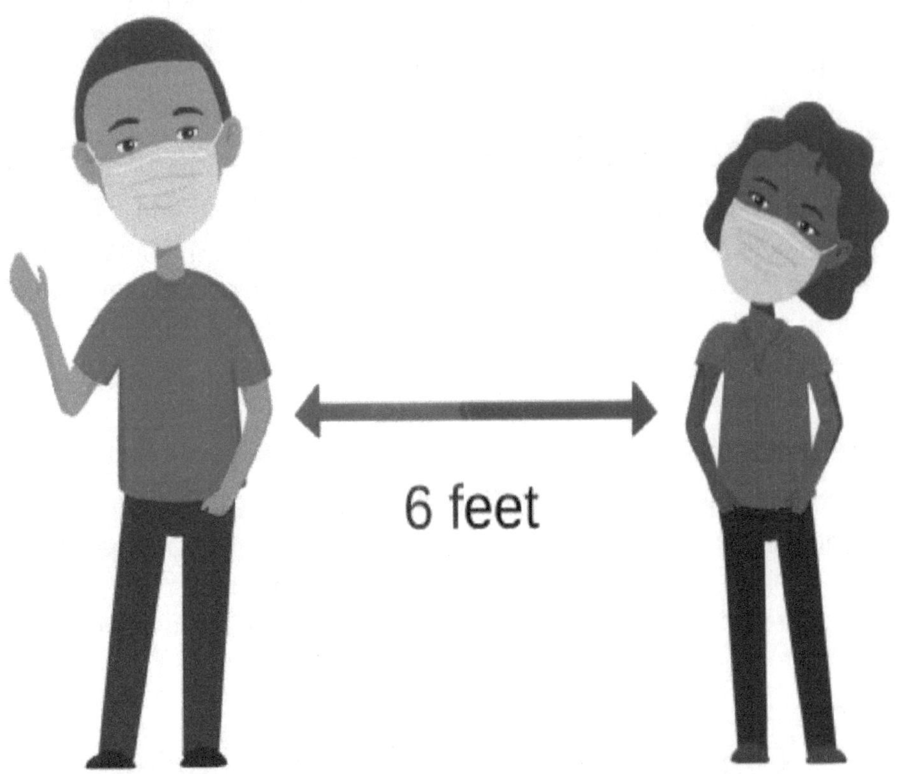


Social distancing (staying 6 feet apart) is the best way to protect yourself. If
you're going to have contact with others, wear a mask and try to stay
outside. We know it's tough. Here are some tips and tricks for common
situations:

* Hug strategically. **Try not to hug at all**, but if it's truly necessary, do
  everything you can to reduce risk. Hugging should be done quickly
  and with faces turned away from each other. Hold your breath
  during the hug and breathe out once you've pulled away.

- **Avoid kissing**. We all want to show some love, but saliva is a huge carrier for COVID-19. This means no kissing - there is just no way to predict who may potentially be sick. A kiss on the top of the head is the safest option if you must.
- **Don't share food or drink**. Finger foods are hosts for virus-carrying fomites!

## Shopping/Dining

- **Grocery shop efficiently**. The grocery store (with a mask and even gloves) is not dangerous if you wipe down your cart and move quickly through the store with your list. (Bringing the whole family is more risky - take some alone time!) Once at home, wash fresh produce (fruits and vegetables) you picked up from the bin with cold running water (not soap or bleach). It is not necessary to wash packaged food.[29]
- While in crowds, **be aware if you are downwind** of or behind others who are not wearing masks, as COVID-19 travels along airflow.
- **Dine out cautiously**. Many restaurants now place tables 6 feet apart, which is great, but it may mean that the people sitting around the tables are still too close to neighboring groups. Taking off masks while eating and drinking creates a high risk of transmission. Enjoy laughter and the fun of gathering while wearing masks! Eat outside and plan your dinner out at a less busy time of day.

## Transportation

- When **using transportation**, take protective measures. Wear a mask over your nose and mouth, don't touch your face, and try to stay 6 feet from others at all times. Wear gloves. Keep your rides short; less than 15 minutes is best. Carry disinfectant wipes for surfaces. Wash your hands or use hand sanitizer before and after your ride.
  - **Ride shares:** Avoid sharing rides with others outside of your home as much as possible. Be sure your driver has a mask on. Sit in the back row, passenger side of the car to create as much space

between you and the driver. Open windows to improve ventilation, wipe down door handles and seat belts, and avoid touching any surfaces. Don't feel obligated to talk to the driver, especially over music.

- **Public transit:** If you're taking public transportation, don't hesitate to move away from passengers who are coughing or appear ill. If you are on a long ride, consider changing positions or cars to avoid long exposures to other passengers. Wear gloves and keep your sunglasses on. Wipe your glasses down when you clean your hands.

## Hotels/Travel

- **Only stay in hotels if you must**. Call beforehand to ask about cleaning procedures and use online check-in and contactless payment. Limit your time spent in shared spaces like lounges, dining areas, and pools. Take the stairs or only ride the elevator with others from your home. Bring your own disinfectant for frequently touched surfaces like light switches, toilets, bathrooms, bedside tables, and lamps.

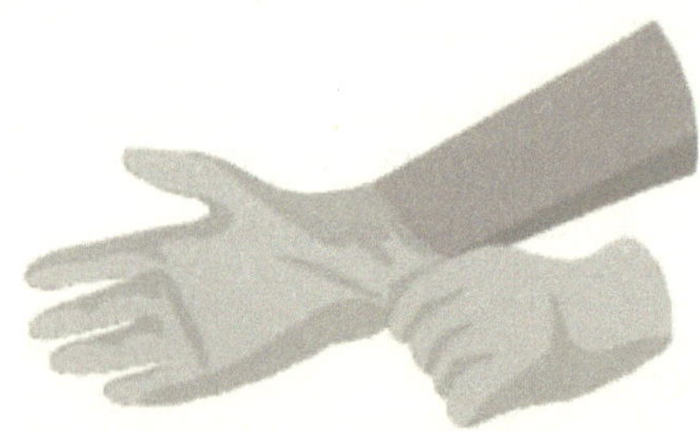

- **Treat airplanes and long train or bus trips like any other form of public transportation.** Mask up, add eye protection and gloves, and avoid close contact and speaking to others. Consider wearing a jacket (or entire outfit) that you remove and bag up to wash when you leave the airport. Check your airline's seating policy to see if they maintain 6 feet between passengers. Wipe down your seat area and seatbelt, bring your own food and water, sit in a window seat, and definitely keep your mask on as other passengers pass you while loading/unloading. This may be the only time you'll want to get on first, and you should still go to the back of the plane. If you can, avoid the restroom.

## To best protect yourself, act as if everyone has COVID-19!

A CDC study reported that **half of surveyed COVID-19 patients couldn't identify who gave them the illness and didn't remember any contacts with symptoms.**[30] This supports the theory that people frequently contract COVID-19 from those who are asymptomatic or have not yet gotten sick - or from surfaces. The CDC estimates that for every 1 case reported, 10 additional COVID-19 cases go undetected.[31] This is why it's so important to avoid large gatherings, wear a mask, wash your hands, and limit contact with people outside of your home.

See more tips for dealing with your environment in the section on Managing Public Areas in Chapter 6: Work!

## Individuals at Higher Risk

## Asthma

People with asthma are at higher risk of being severely infected by COVID-19. Those with an inhaler should carry it with them at all times and use it as directed to maintain healthy airways.

## Smoking/Vaping

Being a current or former cigarette smoker or vaper may increase your risk of severe illness from COVID-19. This is true for all inhaled substances, including marijuana, cocaine, cigars, etc. Take the following actions:

* If you currently smoke, quit. If you used to smoke, don't start again. If you've never smoked, congratulations! Don't ever start.

* It's incredibly hard to quit smoking. Nicotine (and every habit associated with smoking), is deeply addictive. It's not your fault if you can't stop smoking easily. When you quit, it will be the achievement of a lifetime and will probably save your life. Seek out counseling from a healthcare provider AND use FDA-approved medications.[32] These resources can double the chances of quitting smoking.

* For help with quitting smoking, call 1-800-QUIT-NOW or visit smokefree.gov.

* Call your healthcare provider if you have concerns or feel sick. There's a lot of help for quitters of all substances!

## Obesity

Obesity (Body Mass Index [BMI] at or above 30) is one of the many conditions that create a higher risk of severe illness from COVID-19. This is a good time to try a few new healthy recipes. Exercising will help with weight loss and will strengthen the heart and lungs, which will better combat the virus! **Light, enjoyable activity, like walking every day**, is a great way to get outside and start an exercise routine.

## Pregnancy

Women who are pregnant have an increased risk of severe illness from COVID-19.[33] If a pregnant woman develops a fever, cough, trouble breathing, or other symptoms of COVID-19, she should call the doctor, nurse, or midwife to discuss testing and other courses of action.

Pregnant women who are COVID-19 positive might have an increased risk of preterm birth (when the baby is born before the 37th week of pregnancy).[34] Women with more severe sickness, like pneumonia developed from COVID-19, have an increased risk of giving birth prematurely. Preterm birth can be dangerous; in general, babies who are born too early can have serious health problems.

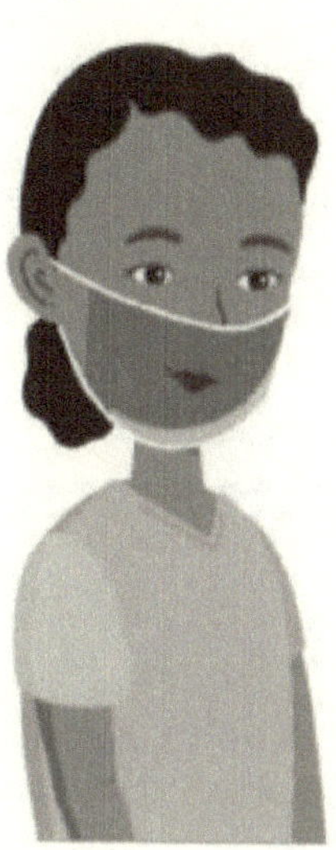

## Babies

It is uncommon for a baby to be infected with COVID-19 while still in the uterus, but it is possible to pass the virus to the baby during childbirth or after the baby is born. Most newborns who test positive for COVID-19 have mild or no symptoms; reports of serious illness are rare. If the mother giving birth is COVID-19 positive, precautions can be taken to lower the risk of transmission. These include:

* Wearing a clear face mask (available online) while with your baby so they can see your face.[35]

* Washing hands and wearing a face covering when within 6 feet of the newborn.

* Wearing a mask when pumping/expressing breast milk.

**NOTE - Never put a face covering on a baby.**

## Maintain your Health

Take care of heart problems, infections, and any ongoing medical issues like cancer, hypertension, or diabetes. It's even more important during this pandemic. Those who take prescription medications regularly should keep an extra month's worth of medication at home. Keeping yourself healthy, even if you have to go to the doctor or dentist, will help keep your immune system strong. If you need to speak to a healthcare professional, try telemedicine; it's a safe way to connect with your medical care team. You can use your phone - FaceTime is allowed!

# Other Ways to Protect Yourself

## Make a Daily Prep Kit

Put together **a bag of the essentials** you'll need as you move through your day: a few masks, a small refillable bottle of hand sanitizer, a pair of cloth gloves, and maybe a pair of plastic gloves. Add some lotion and sunglasses. Remember a packet of disinfecting wipes for surfaces and put a small piece of soap in a baggie. Carry your own water bottle and an extra plastic bag to stash exposed items. Add a small tube of sunscreen and maybe some chapstick since your mask will rub it off your face. Keep your prep kit with your keys and you'll be ready to go.

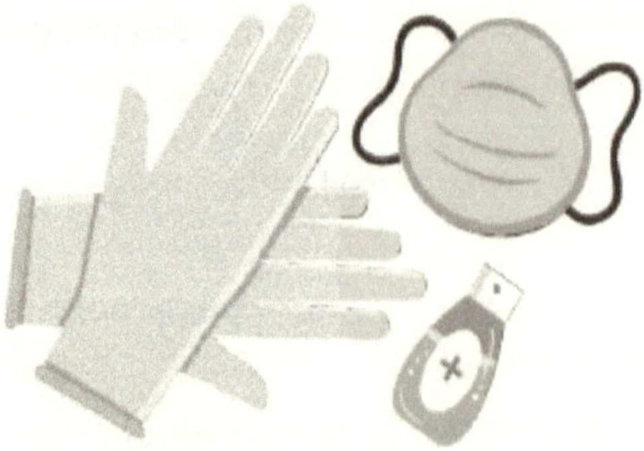

## Make an Illness Prep Kit

Gather up the medication and symptom management items you'll need if you or someone you care for gets sick. Look at Chapter 4: Oh No! to see suggestions. Make a plan, shop while you are healthy, and place what you'll need in a box or in a designated isolation room. Discuss your plan with your family and close friends. Get the numbers of your local ER and health providers, your insurance cards, and contact information for emergency babysitters and keep them in your prep kit. Include gloves, some extra face masks, soap, hand sanitizer, and a printed copy of the charts found in Chapter 8: Track! (and on One Good Turn's website) in case you need them suddenly or late at night.

## Take your Vitals Now

It's a great idea to know what your respiratory rate, oxygen saturation, and temperature are now, while you're well. If you do get sick, you will have a "baseline" for comparison. Look at Chapter 4: Oh No! and Chapter 8: Track! to get started on making your personal medical record.

## Supplements

### COVID-19 and Vitamin D

Supplementing with 1000-2000 IU of vitamin D daily can help to protect you against the effects of COVID-19 in the lungs. Consider a vitamin D supplement, especially if you can't spend time outdoors or have a diet low in vitamin D foods. Very few foods in nature contain vitamin D. Fatty fish (such as salmon, tuna, and mackerel) are good sources. Be careful not to use high daily doses of Vitamin D as too much in the body can become toxic.

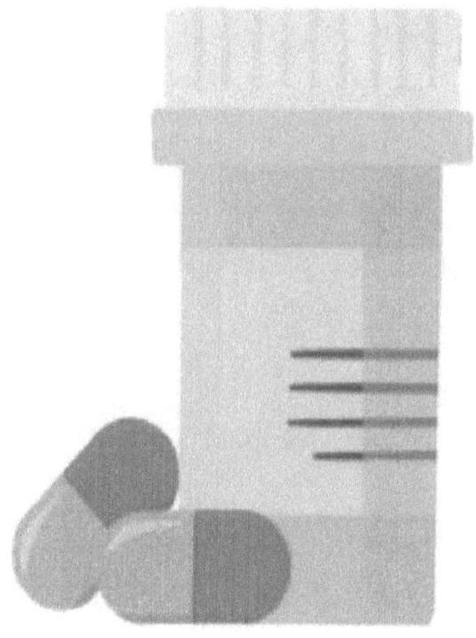

### COVID-19 and Zinc

Supplementing with 10 mg zinc per day can improve your body's ability to fight COVID-19 infection. Food sources of zinc include red meat, poultry, beans, nuts, whole grains, dairy, and fortified cereal. If you get a metallic taste in your mouth after you've been taking zinc supplements for several weeks, take a few days off. Also, check the dose on the package before you buy - many supplements have much higher doses of zinc. You might be able to divide your tablet.

### Vitamin C[36]

65-90 mg of vitamin C daily may be helpful to avoid viral infections, including COVID-19. You can find vitamin C in foods such as bell peppers, fruits, tomatoes, and leafy greens. The higher doses of up to 1000 mg a day are safe but unnecessary unless they help you feel better. While standard doses of vitamin C are generally harmless, high doses can cause a number of side effects, including nausea, cramps, and an increased risk of kidney stones.

### Yearly Flu Vaccine

Remember to get a flu shot as soon as it is available. Many COVID-19 symptoms overlap with flu symptoms, so the immunity created by the flu vaccine will help avoid confusion if you become ill.

## Breathing Exercises

Practicing breathing management exercises for 10-15 minutes twice a day before ever contracting COVID-19 can help increase your lung strength. Take a break between each exercise and slow down or stop if you feel dizzy or out of breath. These exercises should feel good and will become easier with practice.

Belly breathing (using your diaphragm to expand your lungs):

- Sit or lie in a comfortable position with your hands on your belly or the bottom of your ribcage.

* Breathe slowly and steadily in through your nose, expanding your rib cage to fill your lungs entirely with air. Feel a stretch in the back part of your rib cage as your lungs fill with air. This is the largest area of your lungs. Pause, then breathe out through your nose or mouth, feeling your belly and ribs rise and fall with every breath.

Pursed-lips breathing (helps slow your breathing and expand your lungs):

* Breathe in through your nose and fill your lungs, counting as you do.
* Pressing your lips together, breathe out through a small space between your lips, like blowing on a whistle. Count and make the breath out last longer than the breath in (for example, 4 counts in, 6 counts out).

Practicing breathing can increase your lung capacity and will also have a calming effect in these stressful times. For more breathing exercises see the Hesperian Health Guides[37] and the American Lung Association.[38]

## Know Your Exposure Risks

The risk of getting COVID-19 depends on many variables. Consider the space you are in, how many people are nearby, the length of time you stay, and whether those around you are coughing or using loud voices.

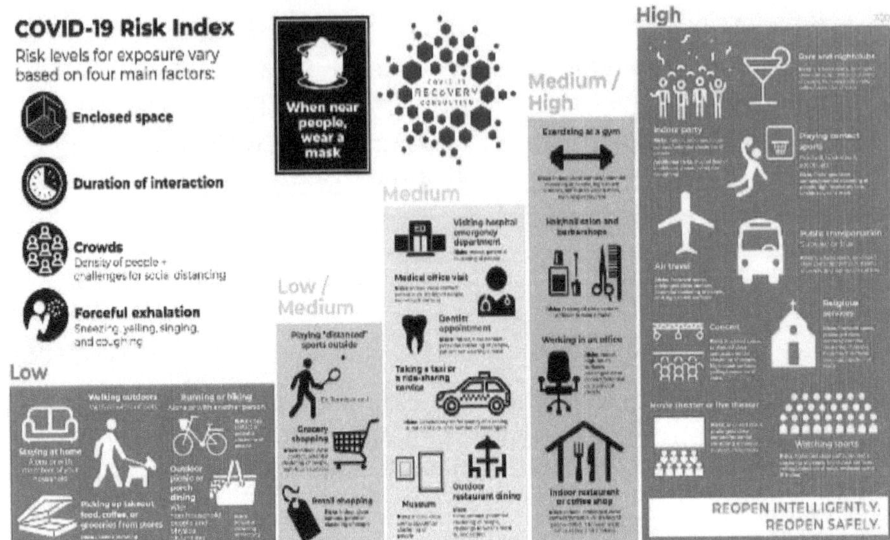




# Mental Health

We know the COVID-19 pandemic can be stressful, especially when the best way to prevent illness is to stay away from others, including your extended family and close friends. **Taking care of your mental health is just as important as taking care of your physical health**. While you must remain physically distanced from others, you must also remain socially connected. Consider reaching out to those you're close to or anyone in your community who may be socially isolated, like an elderly neighbor. We'll get through this together!

## Mental Health in Adults

Reducing COVID-19 related stress and anxiety begins by acknowledging how we feel. Everyone reacts differently to stressful situations, but these are some common signs of stress:

* Changes in sleeping or eating patterns

* Difficulty sleeping or concentrating
* Fear and worry about yourself and loved ones
* Worsening chronic and mental health problems
* Increased withdrawal and isolation
* Increased use of tobacco, alcohol, or other substances

Just as everyone reacts differently to stress, everyone copes differently, too! Here are some practical, healthy ways to cope with the stress and anxiety related to COVID-19:

* **Have a COVID-19 plan**. Know what to do if you are sick or if someone around you is sick. Knowledge is power, and in this case, it can bring a lot of peace of mind!
* **Take care of your body!**
  * Do some light exercise, like taking a walk, stretching, or doing yoga.
  * Try to regularly eat healthy, well-balanced meals.
  * Get plenty of sleep.
  * Avoid excessive tobacco, alcohol, and drug use.
* Make time to unwind. **Do some activities you enjoy!**
* **Connect with others**. Reach out to friends, family, or others in your community. Phone calls or video chats can help you and your loved ones feel less isolated.
* **Take a break from following the news**. Staying informed is really important. However, when broadcasters compete for your attention, they often include anxiety inducing sounds and language, which can increase your stress level. Take regular breaks from all forms of news delivery - phone, TV, and radio - to detach and maintain your own personal outlook.

## Mental Health in Children

Adults aren't the only ones who experience stress and anxiety. Children and teens also feel increased stress during the pandemic as they face their own challenges and react to what they see from the adults around them. To help support your child, try to:

- Talk openly about the COVID-19 pandemic. Be open about what is and is not known about the virus. Reassure your family that it is okay to feel upset or worried.
- Be a role model. Share how you deal with stress. Encourage your child to take breaks, get plenty of sleep, exercise and eat well.
- Limit your family's exposure to the news, including social media and streaming services. Younger children may misinterpret and feel frightened about things they do not understand.
- Spend time with your child doing activities they enjoy.
- Read COVIBOOK, a children's book about COVID-19 that's popular all over the world. Here's a version read in Spanish by a One Good Turn team member.

Mental health is an important part of everyone's overall health and wellbeing. People with preexisting mental health conditions should continue their treatment and be aware of their symptoms. Those with new or worsening symptoms should contact a healthcare provider.

When should I get tested? That question is on everyone's mind. There's more info in the next chapter: TEST! All About Testing.

Good luck! You are a hero for protecting yourself and your family. This is crazy hard, but we will get through it. Reach out to your friends and family, get and give support, and ask for help when you need it. Make a list of your favorite things to do and do one or two of them every day. Give yourself a break. Go for walks. Take care of yourself. You are worth it!

# TEST! ALL ABOUT TESTING

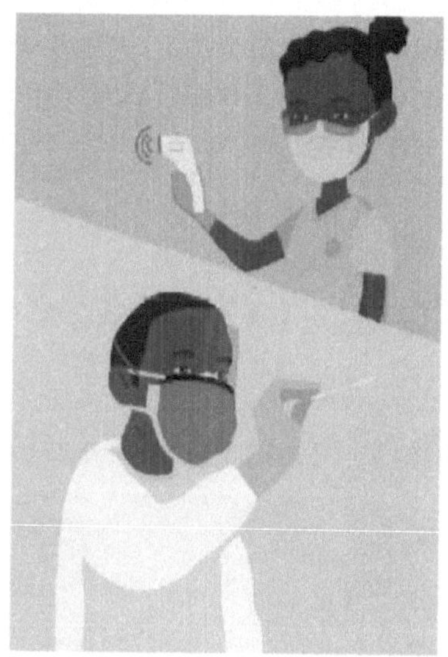

## Chapter 3 Outline

1) COVID-19 Symptoms

2) Should I Get Tested?

3) Frequently Asked Questions

    a) Why do I Have to Get Tested if I Have no Symptoms?

    b) When Should I Get Tested?

    c) How Do I Get Tested for COVID-19?

4) What COVID-19 Tests Are Available?

a) Viral Tests

b) Antibody Tests

c) At-Home Testing

d) "Pooled" Testing

**Testing is tricky.** There are many types of tests and lots of questions about when to get tested and who will pay. Like every aspect of the COVID-19 response, information will change - check the included links and use your healthcare provider and local public health department as resources. The bottom line is that **if you have symptoms that match those of COVID-19, you probably have the virus.** This is a pandemic, after all! Here are the most important basics and a little science to help you make informed decisions.

## COVID-19 Symptoms:

**COVID-19 symptoms vary widely and can range from mild to severe, or a person may have no symptoms at all.** Keep track of any you experience:

* Fever
* Shortness of breath
* Cough (most often a dry cough)
* Sore throat
* Body aches
* Headache
* Fatigue
* Loss of taste
* Loss of smell
* Poor appetite
* Congestion or runny nose
*

Diarrhea, nausea, or vomiting

* Abdominal pain
* Rash on toes or other body parts
* Red eyes

In some people, COVID-19 causes **more severe symptoms like high fever, severe cough, and shortness of breath**, which often indicates pneumonia. See a healthcare provider for any of these symptoms.

Keep an eye on the news and the CDC website for newly added symptoms and updates.

# Should I Get Tested?

**YES - If you have any of the symptoms of COVID-19.**

**YES - If you are a contact.**

You are a contact if you've had **direct, prolonged contact** (more than 15 minutes at less than 6 feet) with someone who has had symptoms OR has tested positive for COVID-19, whether or not you were wearing a mask, even if you don't have symptoms. Examples of close contact situations:

* Household - Someone in your home has tested positive for COVID-19.
* Caregiver - You are taking care of someone with COVID-19.
* Work - Your co-worker in the same work area as you has tested positive for COVID-19.
* School - A classmate who sits near you has tested positive for COVID-19.

Examples of other close interactions listed by the CDC that make you a contact include: direct physical contact with the person (like a hug or a kiss), sharing eating or drinking utensils, and any interaction where a

COVID-19 positive person could have gotten respiratory droplets on you (like a cough or sneeze).

Get tested if you have been **notified by a contact tracer** (usually from the local health department) that you are a contact of someone with COVID-19, whether or not you have symptoms.

**All household members** of a COVID-19 patient should be tested for COVID-19 even if they don't remember having direct contact during the contagious period. Household members can get infected from possible exposure to an infected item or surface in the home that the infected person coughed or sneezed on during the few days **before** the symptoms, if any, started.

## NO - If you are a second-hand contact.

You do not need to get tested if you have had second-hand contact with someone who has tested positive. Second-hand contact means that you are a contact of a contact of a person infected with COVID-19. Examples of second-hand exposure:

- Household - Your spouse's co-worker tested positive (but your spouse needs a test!).
- Work - Someone who works in a different area of the building than you is sick.
- School - Your child's teacher or your roommate's classmate tested positive (and - you got it - your child and roommate would need tests).

## NO - If you want to check for recovery from COVID-19.

The CDC no longer recommends a negative test to end your isolation period if you have had COVID-19. Studies have shown that infected people may still test positive weeks after their illness has resolved, since the viral load that an individual has is different for everyone and the amount of time it takes to rid the body of the virus varies. Turn to Chapter 4: Oh No! for more information on illness and isolation.

# Frequently Asked Questions

## Why do I have to get tested if I have no symptoms?

- You may still have COVID-19 even if you don't show any symptoms, and you can infect your friends and family without realizing it! Asymptomatic cases are dangerous because these individuals are still contagious, and those they infect may have a more severe infection. This is why testing all contacts of those positive for COVID-19 - even if they don't show any symptoms - is so important; having mild symptoms doesn't mean you will pass on a mild form of the disease.

- Testing is how we slow the spread of COVID-19 in our communities. When positive COVID-19 cases are identified, other people who may have been exposed need to be warned and quarantined. Even if you don't get severely ill, it is important to let your contacts know if you are sick.

## When should I get tested?

For a lot of reasons, there is not yet a clear recommendation on this. A diagnostic viral test should be accurate after 3 days or so of symptoms. See specific test details below.

## How do I get tested for COVID-19?

Decisions about testing are made by state and local health departments or healthcare providers. Visit your state[40] CDC website or local[41] health department's website to see the latest local information on testing.

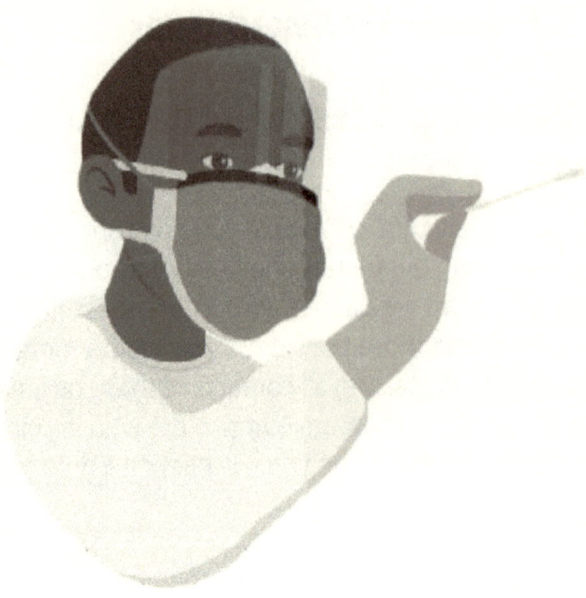

COVID-19 tests are available at no cost at health centers, pharmacies, and community-based testing sites across the U.S. Ask your local health department about free community-based testing sites.[42] The Families First Coronavirus Response Act ensures that COVID-19 testing is free to anyone in the U.S., including the uninsured.

Additional testing sites may be available in your area. **Ask about fees before you get tested. Some health insurance plans that don't consider a test "medically necessary" may charge you for COVID-19 testing**. If you have COVID-19 symptoms and want to get tested, call your healthcare provider or your local public health department first.

## Tips on Testing:

Some COVID-19 tests are more accurate than others, and the best time to get tested during the illness can vary by test as well. **It's possible to get a "false-negative" result, which means that you incorrectly tested negative and actually do have COVID-19**. If the test was done too early in the course of infection, you may eventually test positive for the virus.

**In general, if you test positive, you really do have COVID-19.** If you test negative, there is still a chance you have COVID-19. Use common sense; if you have symptoms, **isolate.** If you know you've been exposed, **quarantine**. See more about how the virus infects you in Chapter 1: What is COVID-19.

## What COVID-19 Tests Are Available?

Two kinds of tests are available for COVID-19: viral tests and antibody tests.[43]

**Viral tests:**

- Test for **current infection.**
- Require a **respiratory system sample**, such as a saliva sample or a swab from the inside of your nose or the back of your throat.

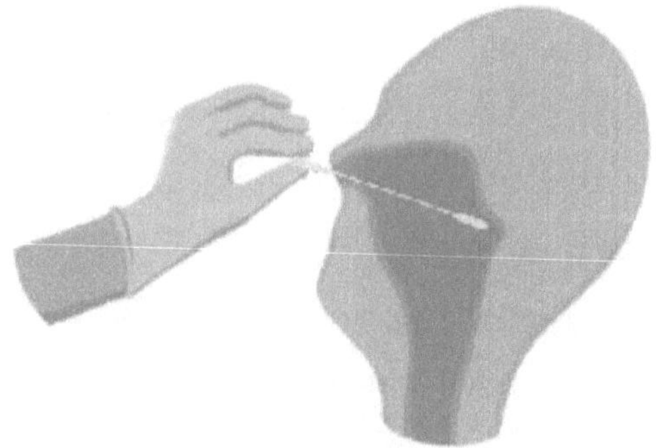

- The **nasal or throat swab** will only be accurate if done correctly. The long swab must be pushed to the back of the nose to test for virus at the place where the nose and the throat connect. Close your eyes and relax - yes, it will be really uncomfortable. It's easier if you can rest the back of your head on a chair or headrest.
- The **saliva sample** is gathered either with a pipette that suctions saliva, a sponge that absorbs saliva, or by having the patient spit directly into a tube.

- Types of viral tests:

- RT-PCR:

    - Tests for viral RNA and DNA
    - Currently the most accurate test
    - Takes several days for results

- Antigen:

    - Tests for specific COVID-19 viral proteins
    - Accurate for positive results (yes, you have COVID-19), but a may be a "false negative"
    - Point-of-care test - results may be available at the testing sit an hour

**Antibody tests:**

- Are also called recovery tests or a serology tests
- Test for **past infection**
- Should NOT be used to check for an active infection
- Require a blood sample
    - fingertip pin-prick
    - blood draw in a lab
- Determine if you've been infected in the past, even if you never showed symptoms
- Detect antibodies called
    - IgM (short-term immune response)
    - IgG (later immune response)

The antibody test checks for an immune response (antibodies) to COVID-19, not for the actual virus. The body doesn't produce antibodies in response to the COVID-19 virus until days to weeks after infection. This is why antibody tests are used to detect past infections, not current infections.

There are a number of antibody tests; some test only for antibodies to the larger coronavirus family of germs and some test just for COVID-19. The more specific tests take longer and are more expensive. Because the coronavirus family includes some of the common cold viruses, if you've recently had a cold you may have a false-positive test for COVID-19 antibodies!

Researchers are working to determine what the immune response to COVID-19 means for the risk of future illness. At first the antibody test was being done in addition to the viral test, but now it is only being done when checking for immunity or **to see if an individual has enough antibodies to donate plasma to severely ill COVID-19 patients**. Researchers hope that antibody tests will provide a more accurate picture of how many people have been infected with and recovered from COVID-19.

## At-Home Testing

The U.S. Food and Drug Administration (FDA) has recently authorized viral tests that let you collect either a nasal swab or a saliva sample at home. You will still need to send your sample to a laboratory for analysis. These at-home tests are an option for easily collecting the samples required for testing without having to travel to a doctor's office or testing site. How you collect and save your sample is the key to getting an accurate result. Follow the instructions carefully!

NOTE - The at-home saliva test costs between $120-$150 and these healthcare providers do not file claims with insurance. The receipt for the COVID-19 test can be submitted to your insurance to be considered for reimbursement.

## "Pooled" Testing

In pooled testing, samples for an entire group or "cohort" of people (for example, a class at school, a shift of co-workers, or a floor of residents in a nursing home) are added together and one test is run on the combined sample. If the test is negative, it means that no one in the cohort has COVID-19. If the test is positive, then each person's specimen will be individually tested while quarantine protocols are started. Often done with saliva (spit) testing, this is a less expensive and more efficient way to screen large groups of people. Look for this testing option in the near future.

So, now you know all about testing. In the next chapter, we'll talk about what to do if you test positive for COVID-19. We'll cover COVID-19 symptoms, your personal COVID-19 treatment plan, and when to seek medical care.

# Chapter 4

# OH NO! I HAVE COVID-19

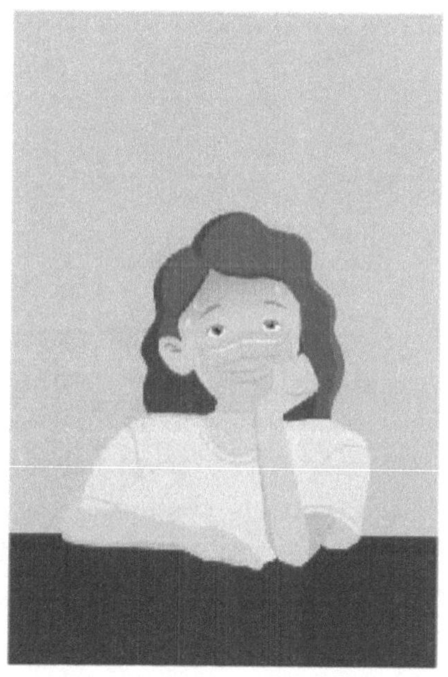

## Chapter 4 Outline

1) Symptoms

2) When to Seek Medical Care

3) Your Personal COVID-19 Treatment Plan

    a) Monitor Your Illness

    b) Your Personal COVID-19 Medical Record

c) Recording Your Vital Signs
    i)  Equipment to Have
    ii) Checking Your Vital Signs

d) Your Symptoms: How Do You Feel?

4) Prevent the Spread of COVID-19

5) Your Response Strategy

a) Medicine

b) Fluids

c) Strengthen Your Body and Immune System

d) Positioning

e) Breathing Exercises

6) When to Go Back To "Normal" Life

a) Immunity

COVID-19 is a brand-new illness with a lot of uncertainty. People can get really sick or have very mild symptoms. While scientists learn more about this new disease, it's hard to know what to do. That's why One Good Turn developed this practical response plan for you to use at home while you're sick. Our goal is to help keep you safe, comfortable, and out of the hospital. Keep this plan close by and share it with others, especially those who are taking care of you. Look through the other chapters of this handbook; all of them will help you get through this illness.

# Symptoms

Symptoms can appear 2-14 days after exposure to COVID-19, or not at all. **You are most contagious during the 2 days before you get symptoms and when you first get them, even if they're mild!** You'll need to isolate for at least 10 days, depending on your situation.

Symptoms vary widely and can range from mild to severe. Watch for common COVID-19 symptoms to appear and keep track of any you experience, including:

- Fever
- Shortness of breath
- Pain when breathing
- Coughing
- Headache
- Fatigue
- Loss of taste or smell
- Sore throat
- Congestion or runny nose
- Diarrhea, nausea, or vomiting
- Rash on toes or other body parts
- Red eyes

As more research is conducted, additional symptoms continue to be identified. Keep an eye on the news and the CDC for symptom updates.[44]

Even if you experience no symptoms or only mild symptoms, you are still contagious and can infect others. Follow isolation guidelines to protect your family and friends.

## When To Seek Medical Care

**Seek emergency medical attention immediately if you show any of these signs:**

- Trouble breathing, including newly increased shortness of breath, or feeling unable to get enough air into your lungs
- Persistent pain or pressure in the chest
- Inability to speak without taking breaths in between words
- Oxygen saturation of 96% or below (95% is the admission threshold

in most hospitals)

* New confusion
* Inability to wake or stay awake
* Lips or face have a blue tint
* Any sudden worsening of pain or other symptoms

This list does not include all possible symptoms. Please call your medical provider if you have any other symptoms that are severe or concerning to you.

Please see <u>Chapter 5</u>: Help! for more information on **caring for kids with COVID-19.**

**Call 911 or your local emergency facility beforehand.** Notify the operator that you are seeking care for COVID-19 related symptoms. **If you can't get through by phone, please go to your medical facility anyway. Health care providers want to care for you even if the phone system is overwhelmed.**

**Day 8 of symptoms is the day when most hospitalizations occur.** Keep a very close eye on your symptoms on days 7-10.

**It is safe to get urgent attention for health needs that don't involve COVID-19.** Call your doctor and seek medical care for both routine health issues and medication refills. Taking care of medical problems as you normally would can prevent big complications later. It's safe to go to the ER for accidents and serious concerns like signs of heart attack, stroke, and pediatric issues.

## Your Personal COVID-19 Treatment Plan

**Isolate yourself** in a separate room from others in your home at the first sign of symptoms, even if you haven't been tested yet. The COVID-19 virus leaves the body from cells in the nose, throat, lungs, eyes, and even feces.

These virus particles get passed on to other people when you cough, sneeze, breathe, or just talk.

**Review your testing options** in Chapter 3: Test! and find out where and how to get tested. Call ahead to schedule your test, if possible, and inform medical office staff of your symptoms - most clinics have a specific set of rules for testing.

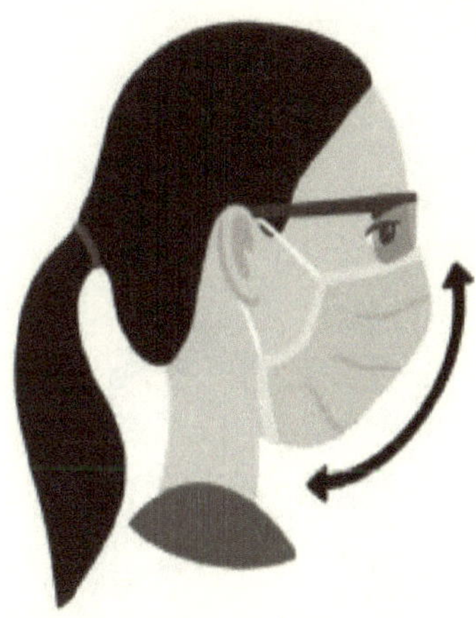

**Wear a mask** and ask others to wear one, too! Wear a mask when exposed to others and whenever you must be outside of your isolation room, even if you are alone, to avoid getting COVID-19 on surfaces around you. Ensure that both your nose and mouth are covered. Masks have been proven to protect you, your family, and any other contacts by limiting the spray of COVID-19 particles when the germs leave your lungs, mouth, throat, and nose.

**Wash your hands** for 20 seconds, or use hand sanitizer for 20 seconds.

- Do this frequently - always after coughing or touching your face and before you touch commonly used items like door knobs, faucets, toilet handles, and public computers.

- Tired of singing the Happy Birthday song? Try the chorus to My Sharona, Staying Alive, Love Shack, Under the Sea, or Bare Necessities. Check the internet[45] for more 20-second songs!

* Keep hand sanitizer with you for any time you can't wash your hands right away.

* You can spread the virus when it gets onto your hands, too. Use disposable gloves, tissues, paper towels, clothing, or plastic bags when touching shared items.

* COVID-19 is found in feces. Yet another reason to wash your hands after using the restroom.

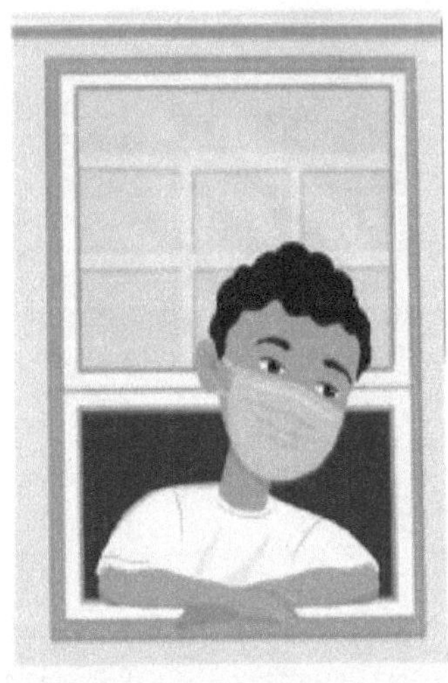

**Practice social distancing.** Keep at least 6 feet between you and anyone else. Remember, masks and social distancing don't replace each other. When you are sick, wear a mask AND keep 6 feet from others at all times.

**Stay home** except to get medical care. Call your medical provider before going to an in-person appointment to get any special instructions for COVID-19 patients, such as waiting in your car instead of the waiting room.

**Tips from One Good Turn:**

* Being outside is okay as long as you're alone or more than 6 feet away from others, AND everybody, including you, is wearing a mask. Any distanced contact with others should last for less than 15 minutes.

- ☀ If you're closer than 6 feet to someone for more than 15 minutes, they will become a contact and will need to quarantine themselves for 14 days per CDC guidelines.
- ☀ Don't eat or drink around others.
- ☀ Remember, you are contagious!

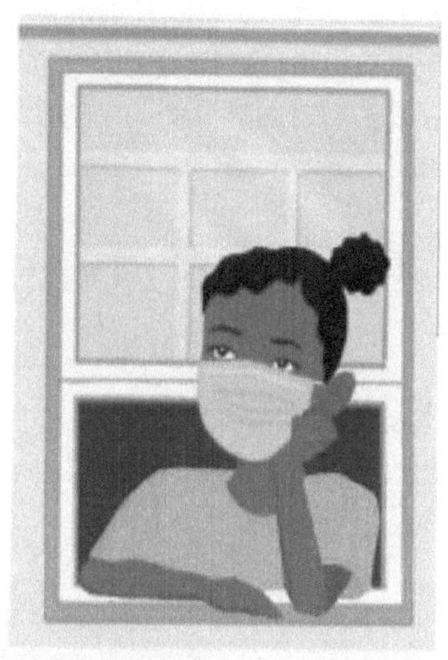

## Monitor Your Illness

By following your symptoms and signs you can take early steps to seek medical care if you need it, and you will have a record of important information for your health care providers.

**Call your doctor's office now to let them know that you are sick.** Even if you don't need to be seen, they will care about how you are doing. You'll get better medical care if your provider is in the loop early. Some prescription medicines might help with your symptoms, especially your cough. Ask about benzonatate capsules, steroids like prednisone or dexamethasone, albuterol or steroid inhalers, and aspirin. Dosing and recommendations will be made by your doctor.

**Fever, cough, and fatigue are the 3 symptoms that predict your risk of getting hospitalized.** Keep an eye on those symptoms.

**Day 8 of symptoms (give or take a few days) is the point in the illness when most people who need to be hospitalized get admitted.** Watch your symptoms closely at this time.

**If you feel fine but have tested positive, you are still contagious.** Many people have no or very few symptoms but still have to isolate (stay away from others) for at least 10 days. It's so hard, but so important. The only way to end this pandemic and prevent serious illness for others is to stop the spread of COVID-19. Keep track of the days of your illness so you know clearly when to stop your isolation - more on that below.

## What Should Your Personal COVID-19 Medical Record Include?

**Your medical information**: List all the basics, including your medical history and any prescription medication, over-the-counter medication, and supplements. Include any allergies.

**Your risk factors**: These include obesity, diabetes, asthma, cancer, hypertension, and heart disease, as well as being Black or Hispanic.

Use the chart in <u>Chapter 8</u>: Track! Here's an example:

| Full Name | | Current Medical | |
| --- | --- | --- | --- |
| Age | | Conditions | |
| Height | | Current | |
| Weight | | Medication | |
| Date and Time Symptoms Began | | Allergies | |

| Higher Risk Categories (Check all that apply and Provide additional information if necessary) | | | |
| --- | --- | --- | --- |
| Hypertension | | Malignancy | |
| Diabetes | | Postpartum (<6 weeks) | |
| Obesity | | Pregnancy (if yes, trimester) | |
| Asthma | | Liver Disease | |
| Heart Conditions | | Chronic neurological or neuromuscular disease | |
| Lung Conditions | | Immunodeficiency, including HIV | |
| Other(s), please specify | | | |

**Your medications**: Make a list of the medicines you take (both regular medications and what you're taking for COVID-19 symptoms).

- Record the time and date when you take each dose (it's hard to remember this when you feel awful).

- Print this chart (in Chapter 8: Track!) as many times as you need and record all medicine you take until you've recovered. You can also find and print this medical chart at onegoodturn.org.

Medicine Tracking Chart: Use this chart to record the date, time, and dose of your medications.

| Date | Time | Medicine | Dose |
|------|------|----------|------|
|      |      |          |      |
|      |      |          |      |
|      |      |          |      |
|      |      |          |      |
|      |      |          |      |
|      |      |          |      |
|      |      |          |      |
|      |      |          |      |
|      |      |          |      |
|      |      |          |      |
|      |      |          |      |
|      |      |          |      |
|      |      |          |      |

Nobody knows your situation better than you! Having this important information written down now will keep you prepared and ready to act if you need to seek care.

## Recording Your Vital Signs

Vital signs are physical findings described by numbers. Changes in your vitals signs predict worsening or improving illness. That's why vital signs are checked at every medical appointment. Having some equipment will help you monitor your vital signs at home. These devices can be shared among family and friends, but only after they are disinfected.

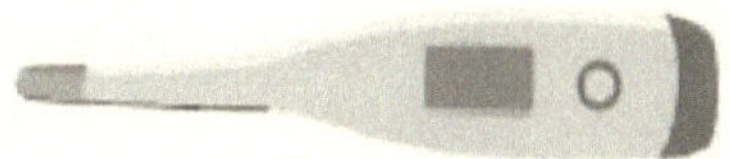

**Equipment to have on hand, if possible:**

Digital thermometer:

   * Disinfect the thermometer before and after using it.

Fingertip oxygen saturation monitor (pulse oximeter):

   * These are available at a pharmacy or online.

If you can't get these supplies, it's okay. You can keep track of your symptoms - which are just as important - without any special tools. We'll discuss that next.

**Checking your vital signs:**

**Temperature:**

   * Pay special attention if your fever is 100.4 degrees or higher because a high fever is a sign of worsening illness.[46]
   * If you have an elevated temperature (above 99.4), check it at least every 4 hours. (A normal temperature is 98.6 degrees.)
   * Keep track of your fever even if you're taking fever-lowering medications.
   * Often it takes 3 measurements to get a good average reading, especially with forehead thermometers.
   * NOTE - If you've been outside in the heat, your temperature may be a bit high. Step inside, wait a few minutes to cool off, and try again.

**Oxygen saturation (O2 Saturation %):** Oxygen saturation monitors are little machines powered by AAA or AA batteries. They clip onto your finger and give you a basic oxygen level reading in a few seconds.

❋ To check your O2 saturation, sit down and relax.

1. Squeeze open the monitor and you will see a tiny red flashing li
2. Put your palm down on a surface, slip the monitor onto the end
   second or third finger with the number side up (over your finge
   the pad of your finger over the red light inside. It will not hurt.
3. Wait several seconds and you will see 2 numbers. Both will be la
   your pulse (heart rate) and your O2 saturation (the percentage c
   your blood).

❋ Your O2 saturation should be above 96% - it will most likely be 97%
or 98%.

❋ Take a "baseline" O2 saturation reading before you feel ill so you
have a comparison for later.

❋ Keep a written record of your results; the machine does not store
them.

❋ If your O2 saturation percent drops to 95%, seek medical care.

❋ If your breathing suddenly gets worse or more painful, go to the
emergency room. Call first if you can.

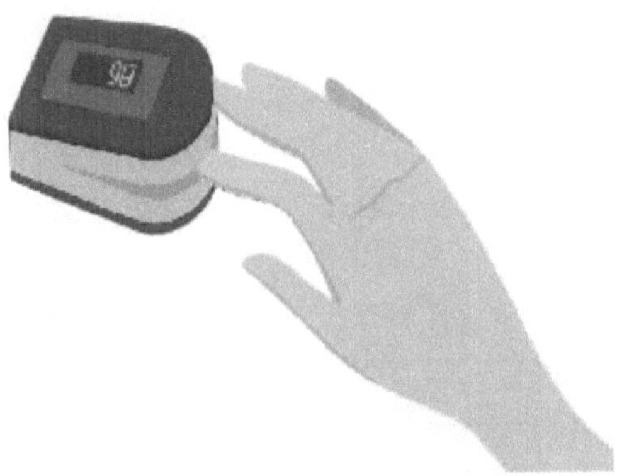

**Breaths per minute (Respiratory Rate or RR):** If you are having trouble
breathing, seek medical care, whatever your respiratory rate is.

❋ No special equipment is needed, just a person to observe your breathing and a watch with a second hand!

* Count the number of breaths you take in 30 seconds and multiply that number by 2 (a breath is one inhale and one exhale).

* It's hard to measure your own respiratory rate. If there is someone else around, have them count your breathing for you.

* A respiratory rate of 18 or less is normal for adults. If your respiratory rate is more than 20 breaths per minute and you feel breathless, seek medical care.

* Kids breathe much faster than adults. You can find information about this in Chapter 8: Track! Call your family doctor right away if your child has trouble breathing.

You can use OGT's vital sign tracking chart to keep track of your results. This chart is in Chapter 8: Track!

| Record the following signs to the best of your ability. (Print this page twice and record signs for 10 days) | | | | | | | | | | |
|---|---|---|---|---|---|---|---|---|---|---|
| Signs | Day 1 AM | Day 1 PM | Day 2 AM | Day 2 PM | Day 3 AM | Day 3 PM | Day 4 AM | Day 4 PM | Day 5 AM | Day 5 PM |
| Fever > 100.4 | | | | | | | | | | |
| Adult O2 Sat % | | | | | | | | | | |
| Child O2 Sat % | | | | | | | | | | |
| Adult Respiratory Rate (breaths per minute) | | | | | | | | | | |
| Child Respiratory Rate (breaths per minute) | | | | | | | | | | |
| Blood Pressure | | | | | | | | | | |

## Your Symptoms: How Do You Feel?

Most care plans for COVID-19 are based on symptom type, severity, and duration. **Feelings of deep fatigue or exhaustion, confusion, weakness, being feverish, and difficulty breathing are all reasons to seek medical care**. It's hard to remember the severity or duration of your symptoms when you feel bad or are under stress; keeping a record will provide important information to health care workers and help you make informed decisions if you need to seek medical care. Also, tracking your symptom improvement will help you determine when you can end your 10 day (minimum) isolation period (see "When to Go Back to 'Normal' Life" below).

Keep a record of your symptoms (the way you feel) day by day. Use our symptom tracker in Chapter 8: Track!

| Record your symptoms on a scale of 1-5: 1 being normal & 5 being severe. (Print this page twice and record symptoms for 10 days) | | | | | | | | | | |
| --- | --- | --- | --- | --- | --- | --- | --- | --- | --- | --- |
| symptom | Day 1 AM | Day 1 PM | Day 2 AM | Day 2 PM | Day 3 AM | Day 3 PM | Day 4 AM | Day 4 PM | Day 5 AM | Day 5 PM |
| Subjective Fever (Y/N) | | | | | | | | | | |
| Cough | | | | | | | | | | |
| Shortness of Breath/ Dyspnea | | | | | | | | | | |
| fatigue/ Malaise/ Myalgias | | | | | | | | | | |
| Sore throat | | | | | | | | | | |
| Nasal Congestion | | | | | | | | | | |
| Diarrhea/ Nausea/ Vomitting | | | | | | | | | | |
| Other Symptoms | | | | | | | | | | |

## Prevent the Spread of COVID-19

As much as possible, stay in a separate room away from other people in your home. Use a separate bathroom as well, and cover your coughs and sneezes.

If you must share a bedroom:

- Open windows and turn on fans to circulate air.
- Place your bed away from room vents so that COVID-19 will not be

spread to others by air flowing across you.

* Avoid sharing a bed with others. Sleep head to toe if space is tight.
* Keep beds at least 6 feet apart, if possible.
* Hang a curtain or other physical divider to separate your bed from others - a plastic shower curtain will work.

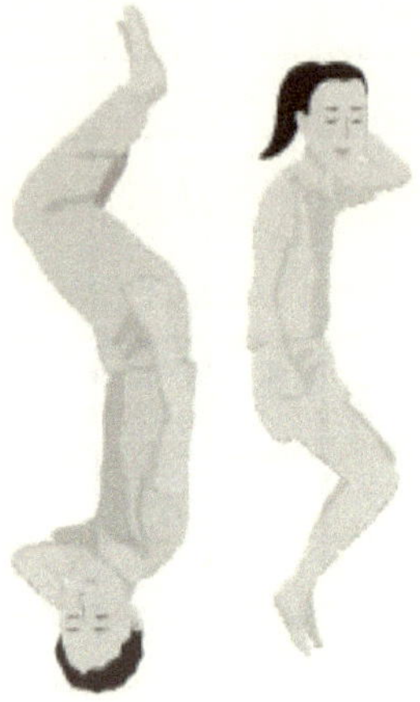

If you must share a bathroom:

* Disinfect any surfaces touched after each use.
* Put a long-acting bleach tablet into the toilet tank.
* Close the toilet lid before flushing to minimize spray from the toilet bowl. COVID-19 is found in feces, and particles do spray into the air.

Meals:

* Don't help prepare food.
* Stay out of the kitchen. No doing dishes for you!
* Eat separately from others, preferably in your isolation room.
* Try to use disposable plates, utensils, and cups. Bag them up in your own covered trash can. When it is full, tie the bag closed and make sure it goes directly outside.

Laundry:

- Your towels, sheets, and clothes can go in a regular washer and dryer.
- Do your own laundry if possible. Wear a mask and gloves when handling dirty items.
- Handle items gently to avoid releasing COVID-19 particles into the air.

# Your Response Strategy

**Those who get sick from the COVID-19 virus feel terrible**. It can be much worse than the flu, with a really high fever, an awful cough, and bad chest pain and body aches. People feel exhausted, too. Stay ahead of symptoms by taking medicine regularly and drinking lots of fluids. It's easier to keep a fever down and keep a cough settled than it is to break a fever or a terrible coughing spell. The breathing and positioning techniques below are also really important ways to keep lung function at its best.

# Medicine

Medication may help improve your symptoms and may keep your COVID-19 infection from getting worse, but none of these medicines are cures. Right now, the only cure is time!

Here are some medications you can take that can **make the infection less severe**:

- Vitamin D can help prevent pneumonia.
  - Take a 20,000 IU dose daily for 3 days, then take 2000 IU daily until you're better. IU stands for International Units and is different from mgs (milligrams). IUs are dosing units for certain vitamins, including vitamin D, and will be listed on the label of the bottle.
  - NOTE - Do not take more vitamin D than the doses listed here!

* Zinc can help prevent COVID-19 from entering your cells.
    * Take a 20 mg dose daily for 2 weeks or until you're better.
* Vitamin C can help to prevent and fight COVID-19.[47]
    * Formulations vary, so follow package dosing up to 1000 mg daily.
    * Vitamin C is also available as an "immune complex" with vitamin D, zinc, and other vitamins and minerals.

Here are some medications you can take to **lower your fever**:

* Acetaminophen (Tylenol, paracetamol):
    * The adult dosing is 650-1000 mg every 4-6 hours. (The long-acting dose is higher and that's fine!)
    * NOTE - Do NOT take more than 4000 mg of acetaminophen per day.
* Alternating doses of ibuprofen (Advil, Motrin):
    * **If acetaminophen alone does not control your fever, you can alternate it with ibuprofen. Take one or the other every 4 hours.**
    * The adult dosing is 600 mg every 8 hours.
    * Children's dosing is based on age and weight. Check the packaging for dosing instructions.
    * NOTE - Ibuprofen can cause stomach irritation (gastritis). To protect your stomach, take ibuprofen with food and/or add an acid blocker, like famotidine (Pepcid). Adults and children weighing 40 kgs (90 lbs) or more can take 20 mg 2 times per day, in the morning and at bedtime, for up to 6 weeks. Review the label for dosings for this and other acid blocker medications.

Here are some medications you can take to **improve your cough and congestion**:

* Guaifenesin (Mucinex, Robitussin):

- These medications loosen mucus.
- The adult dosing (immediate release) is 100-400 mg every 4 hours.
- The adult dosing (extended release) is 600-1200 mg every 12 hours.
- NOTE - Do NOT take more than 2.4 g or 2400 mg of guaifenesin per day.

* Dextromethorphan (Delsym, Robitussin DM, Nyquil):
  - These medications are cough suppressants, typically used at night.
  - The adult dosing is 10-20 mg orally every 4 hours.
  - Do not take more than 120 mg of dextromethorphan per day.
  - NOTE - Do NOT give dextromethorphan to a child younger than 4 years old.

* Cough drops:
  - These can soothe irritation in the nose and throat.
  - Choose your favorite flavors.

* Pseudoephedrine (Sudafed):
  - The adult dosing is 30-60 mg every 4 hours, or less as needed for nasal congestion.
  - Children's dosing is based on age and weight. Check the packaging for dosing instructions.

NOTE - A steam humidifier can help keep your throat and upper airways moist and comfortable. If warm steam is used, keep the machine safely away from your sleeping area to avoid burns. Try filling a bathroom sink with hot water and adding a few drops of an essential oil of your choice (like eucalyptus). Sit down, drape a towel over your head and the sink, breathe deeply, and relax for a few minutes.

## Fluids

Drink lots of fluids. Staying hydrated will help to keep any fluids in your lungs loose and easier to cough up. Honey lemon tea and savory broths with garlic have antiinflammatory effects as well. Being well-hydrated will also help you feel generally better. The **athlete's rule:** Keep your pee light yellow! Any clear (non-alcoholic) fluids that sound good to you are fine.

Here's a calculation for hydration: As a baseline, drink ½ your body weight in ounces of water daily. So, if you weigh 200 lbs you need 100 oz, or at least 12 cups, to stay hydrated. If you are sick, you'll need to drink up to ⅔ of your body weight in ounces - in this example, that's about a gallon (128 oz) of fluids. Your body needs fluids to fight off infection and make up for fluid losses from coughing, fever, and the effort of breathing. Keep a full glass of water and whatever tastes best to you by your bed. Take a big sip every 5 minutes or at least 2 cups every hour while you are awake. A steady intake of fluids will work better than occasionally chugging down a bottle. Pedialyte, sports drinks, effervescent vitamin packets, or a slice of lemon in your water can help with taste and hydration.

## Strengthen Your Body and Immune System

A strong immune system helps you fight off and recover from COVID-19.

- Eat healthy foods like fatty fish, fruits, and vegetables - include your favorite comfort foods!
- Eat foods that strengthen your immune system like ginger, garlic, and tumeric.
- Rest as much as you need to - get at least 7-8 hours of sleep each

night.

- Spend at least 15 minutes in the sun each day to help your body make vitamin D (the darker your skin or the older you are, the more time in the sun you need).

- Don't smoke; avoid drinking too much alcohol. See Chapter 2: Yikes! for information on quitting smoking.

## Positioning

Move around to keep your lungs full of air. Position changes can help with breathing. The largest part of your lungs are on the back side of your body, so when you lie on your stomach (prone) your lungs can get more oxygen. Sleep on your stomach if possible. Put a few pillows under your hips when you are prone.

You may feel like all you can do is lie in bed, but it actually takes more effort to breathe while lying flat! Try resting in different positions and keep moving around. Set up a routine to remind yourself to move. For example, get up for 10 minutes after every 30-minute episode of your favorite TV show. Gentle movements can really help with breathing. Try walking around your room, raising your arms over your head, and slowly stretching and twisting your upper body.

Postural drainage moves fluid away from the lungs. Spend several minutes in each position. Start as soon as you have any breathing symptoms.

- **Back**: Lie with 2-3 pillows under your hips so that your stomach is higher than your chest. Rest your arms by your side and breathe in through your nose and out through your mouth. Try to breathe out for longer than you breathe in.

- **Sides**: Lie on your side with 2-3 pillows under your stomach so that your chest is lower than your hips. Breathe in through your nose and out through your mouth. Try to breathe out for longer than you breathe in. Switch sides.

- **Stomach**: Lie on your front with 2-3 pillows under your stomach to raise it above your chest. Rest your arms by your head and breathe in through your nose and out through your mouth. Try to breathe out for longer than you breathe in.

## Breathing Positions

**1. 30 minutes - 2 hours: laying on your belly**
1. 30 minutos - 2 horas: acostado sobre su estómago (boca abajo)

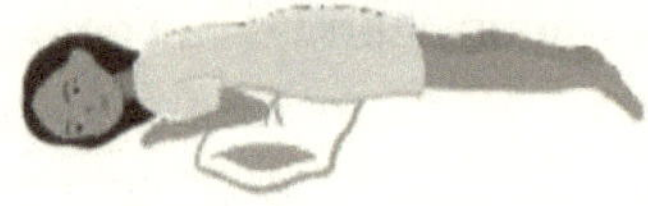

**4. 30 minutes - 2 hours: lying on your left side**
4. 30 minutos - 2 horas: acostado sobre su lado izquierdo

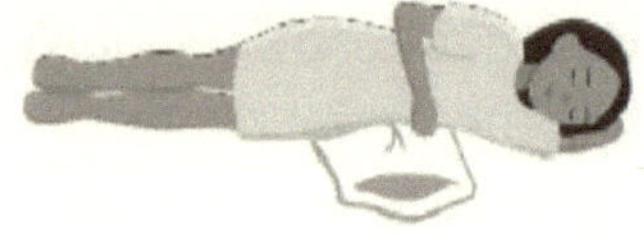

**2. 30 minutes - 2 hours: laying on your right side**
2. 30 minutos - 2 horas: acostado sobre su lado derecho

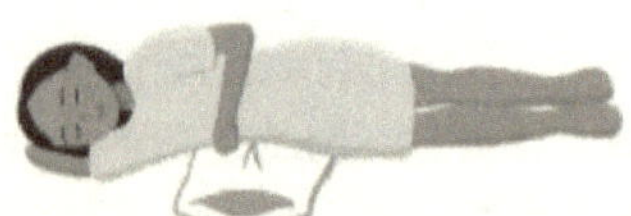

**Then back to Position 1. Lying on your belly!**
Luego, vuelva a la posición 1. (Acostado sobre su estómago (boca abajo!)

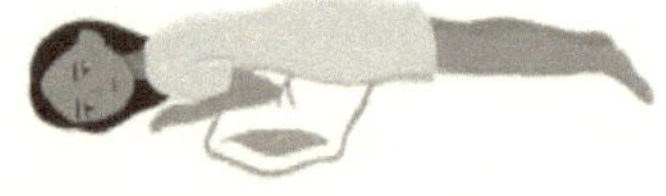

**3. 30 minutes - 2 hours: sitting up**
3. 30 minutos - 2 horas: sentado

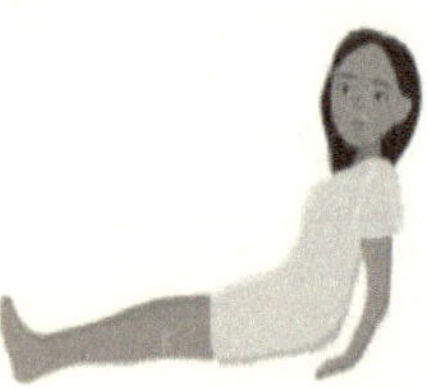

If you have a lot of congestion in your lungs, seek the advice of a doctor - you may need further evaluation.

## Breathing Exercises

Start breathing exercises now, even if you don't have shortness of breath or painful breathing. A breath is 1 inhale and 1 exhale. This will help prevent fluid from collecting in the lungs. Do these breathing exercises for 10-15 minutes, at least 2-4 times a day. The more you practice, the easier they will become and the better they will make you feel. For all exercises, breathe in through your nose. It cleans, warms and moistens the inhaled air. Breathing exercises are also calming and can help with anxiety.

Feel your breathing - also called belly or diaphragm breathing:

- Sit or lie down in a comfortable position. Put your hands on the bottom of your ribcage, where you can feel your ribs and your belly.
- Breathe in through your nose and feel your entire lungs fill with air in both the front and the back. Breathe out through your nose or mouth. Feel how your belly and ribs rise as you breathe in and fall as you breathe out.

Pursed-lips breathing - this helps slow your breathing and expand your lungs:

- Breathe in through your nose and fill your lungs, counting as you inhale.
- Pressing your lips together, breathe out through a small space between your lips, like blowing out a candle. Count and make the breath out last longer than the breath in (for example, 4 counts in, 6 counts out).

Deep breathing - this opens the chest and can help loosen congestion in your lungs:

- Breathe slowly and gently when breathing deeply.
- Take a slow, deep breath through your nose.
- Hold your breath for 2-3 seconds before gently breathing out, like a sigh. Do this 3-5 times.

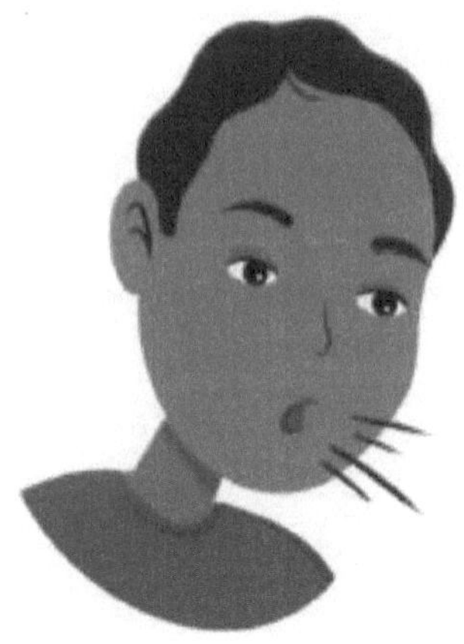

Huffing - this helps move congestion out of the lungs:

- Breathe in normally and then push your breath out quickly and forcefully through your mouth until your lungs feel empty.
- Open your mouth wide. Your breath going out will make a "huff" sound.
- Repeat this several times. If you hear a crackling noise when you huff, gentle coughing may help you clear the congestion.

For more breathing exercises see the Hesperian Health Guides[48] and the American Lung Association.[49]

## When To Go Back To "Normal" Life

- **People with COVID-19 who have symptoms** may discontinue isolation under the following conditions:[50]
  - At least 10 days have passed since symptom onset **and**
  - At least 24 hours have passed since resolution of fever without the use of fever-reducing medications **and**
  - Other symptoms have improved.
- **People who have a positive respiratory test for COVID-19 but**

**never develop COVID-19 symptoms** may discontinue isolation when:

> • At least 10 days have passed since the confirmed test **and**

> • NO symptoms have developed.

- **Negative tests are no longer recommended to demonstrate recovery.**

## Immunity

Nobody knows if we develop COVID-19 immunity or how long it might last last. While the body usually makes some protective antibodies after getting COVID-19, it's unknown whether all patients develop any long-term protective response. If you've had COVID-19, you can still get it again. Keep wearing your mask and following daily prevention practices even after you recover! Some people relapse, so keep an eye out for new or returning symptoms for several weeks.

Yay! You made it! and you have a great story to tell. According to the CDC and WHO, once you recover you can safely go back to the "new normal" of interaction with social distancing and masks. This includes work, play, and family life. If you have successfully isolated and kept from getting sicker, you did your job!

Remember to **get a flu shot** as soon as it is available - you won't want to get sick again any time soon. Many COVID-19 symptoms overlap with flu symptoms, so the immunity created by the vaccine will help avoid confusion should you become ill.

Now that you're well, **you can donate convalescent plasma** to help other COVID-19 patients. This heroic act is just like giving blood! Check with your local blood bank to sign up. Then, with a negative COVID-19 PCR test (swab or saliva) and maybe an antibody test (blood test, pinprick or lab test), a small bag of your blood is drawn from an IV in your arm. In a lab, the blood is "spun down." Red blood cells, heavier because of the iron they contain, move to the bottom of the bag, leaving the clear fluid called plasma. Your plasma has your antibodies in it: valuable cells that your body made while fighting off COVID-19. When this plasma is given by vein to a person hospitalized with COVID-19, it is proven to help their immune system fight off the cytokine storm of COVID-19 so they can recover, too.[51] What a gift!

Okay, you know what to do if YOU get sick, so now let's talk about what to do if a loved one, friend, or roommate gets the virus. In the next chapter, we'll go over how to take care of someone who has tested positive for COVID-19.

# HELP! I'M TAKING CARE OF SOMEONE WITH COVID-19

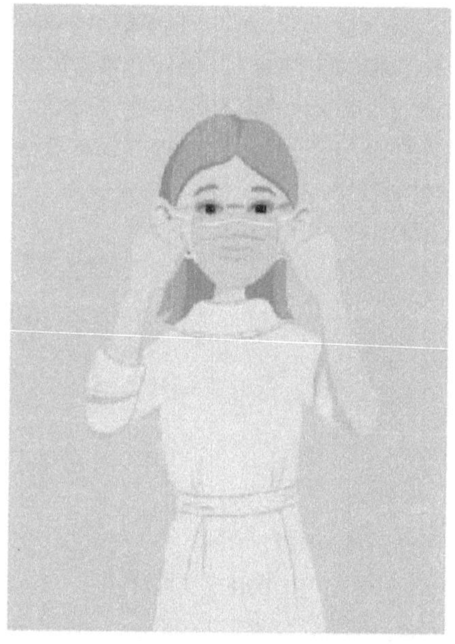

## Chapter 5 Outline

1) Getting Started
2) Isolate the Sick Person
3) Protecting Others in the House
   a) Keeping Yourself (the Caregiver) Safe

i) How to Use Your Personal Protective Equipment

4) Your Role as the Caregiver

5) COVID-19 and Children

a) What Should I do if my Child has Symptoms?

b) Multisystem Inflammatory Syndrome in Children

6) When to Go Back to "Normal" Life

a) Immunity

CONGRATS! YOU ARE NOW A HEALTHCARE PROVIDER! Caring for someone who is sick with COVID-19 is not easy. Here are some tips for how to provide care for a sick person while still protecting yourself and others in your household. **Seek medical care for your "patient" if you start to feel overwhelmed**. Explore your care options now, before you need them. Establish contact with your health care provider and stay in touch with your personal support system. Remember that you are now in a high-risk situation. Use the recommendations in <u>Chapter 2</u>: Yikes! to protect yourself.

## Getting Started

Refer to our other chapters in the Corona Care Handbook to develop a "plan of care" depending on how your patient feels. Read <u>Chapter 4</u>: Oh No! for medicine, symptoms, guidelines, and resources on how to care for patients with mild to severe symptoms. You will need the Track! and Yikes! chapters as you monitor the sick person while still protecting others in your home. Print the Track! symptom tracker if possible.

## Isolate The Sick Person

Isolate the sick person from others in your home at the first sign of symptoms, even if they haven't been tested yet. The patient should stay in a separate room away from other people in the home as much as possible. They should also use a separate bathroom if there is one available. Have your sick person wear a mask for the short times when they may be around others in the house, and whenever they leave their room, to avoid getting COVID-19 virus on surfaces in your home. Make sure their nose AND mouth are covered at all times.

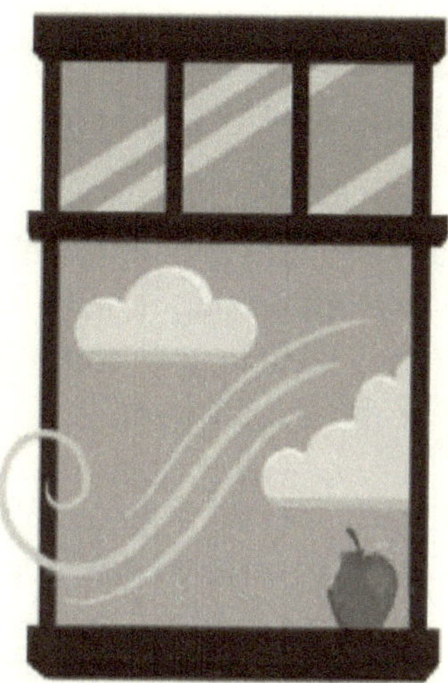

Make a comfortable sick room (an "isolation room") where the person with COVID-19 can spend their time separated from everyone else. A room down a hallway or away from the main living area would be great. Bring your patient's comfort things into the room; they will be there for a while! If there is an air conditioning return vent that takes air up from the room (not the one that blows out), cover it up. The room should have:

* Outlets for phones/electronic devices
* A TV and/or computer, if possible
* A window or outside door for ventilation
* A pitcher of water and a glass just for the patient
* Tissues and paper towels
* Wipes and surface cleaning supplies
* Personal hygiene supplies like a toothbrush, face wipes, a hairbrush, etc. (Think like you are packing for a trip.)
* A designated bathroom just for the COVID-19 positive person, if

possible (If not, keep lots of cleaning supplies in the bathroom.)

* A trashcan lined with a garbage bag
* A hamper for bedding and clothes
* Extra blankets, pillows, washcloths, and towels
* A cooler (optional)
* And any other items you think of as you get the room set up

NOTE - If you're in a large household and believe more people may be infected by your patient, one option might be to find out if there's a COVID-19 isolation facility available in your community. They're usually free and run by the local health department.

The sick person should stay home except to get medical care. Call your medical provider before going to an in-person appointment for any special instructions for COVID-19 patients.

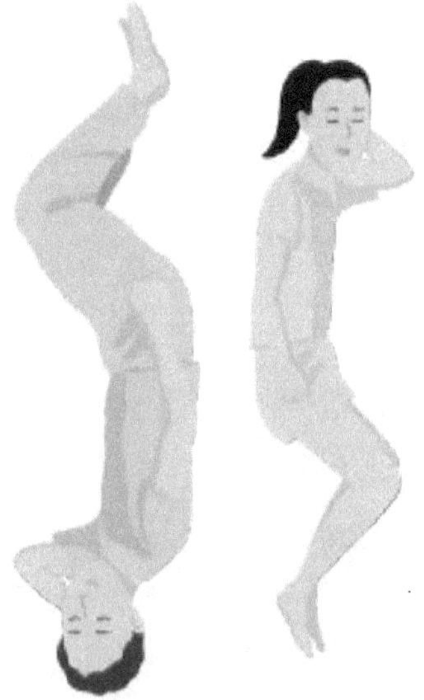

If the patient must share a bedroom:

* Hang a curtain or shower curtain, or set up a physical divider, to

separate the sick person's bed.

- Open windows and turn on fans to circulate air.
- Keep the sick bed away from room vents so airflow doesn't spread the virus.
- Keep 6 feet between beds, if possible.
- If space is really tight, sleep head to toe.

If the patient must share a bathroom:

- Have your patient wear a mask in the bathroom.
- Disinfect any surfaces touched after each use.
- Put a long-acting bleach tablet into the toilet tank.
- Close the toilet lid before flushing to minimize spray from the toilet bowl. COVID-19 is found in feces, and particles do spray into the air!

Meals

- Your patient should not help prepare food and should stay away from the kitchen.
- Use disposable plates, utensils, and cups - it will make things easier! Your person can put them in the trash in their isolation room; the full bag goes directly outside.
- Leave a lined trash bag in the sick person's room. Use disposable gloves and wear a mask when removing garbage bags or handling trash.
- If washing dishes, use a dishwasher or hot water and soap. Wear gloves while handling used dishes and wash your hands for at least 20 seconds immediately afterwards.
- Your patient should eat separately from others. It's best for them to eat in their isolation room; the time they spend eating without a mask is high-risk for others.
- When you bring food to your person, leave it at the door and don't

stay with them while they eat. This may sound really lonely, but you need to protect yourself and others in your household. Eating is a high-risk activity. FaceTime during family meals!

Laundry

* Contaminated towels, sheets, and clothes can go in a regular washer and dryer.
* Wear a mask and gloves (if possible) when handling dirty items.
* Handle items gently to avoid spreading COVID-19 particles into the air.
* Don't share personal items like bedding, dishes, utensils, phones, or towels.

Going outside is okay as long as:

* Your patient is alone or more than 6 feet apart from others.
* Everybody wears a mask.
* Distanced contact with others is for less than 15 minutes.
* All doors and surfaces your patient may have touched are wiped down.

## Protecting Others in the House

* Improve the ventilation of your house as much as possible - open windows and screened doors and turn on fans.

- Cleaning

  - Disinfect reusable items (for example, thermometers) between uses with 70% ethyl alcohol.

  - Disinfect frequently touched surfaces (for example, door knobs or bathroom surfaces) with disinfecting wipes or sprays. You can make your own disinfecting solution using household bleach with a sodium hypochlorite concentration of 5%-6%, which is effective against coronaviruses.[52] Dilution is required for safe, appropriate use. See Chapter 2: Yikes! for dilution instructions. Wear gloves when handling bleach!

  - Other EPA-approved cleaners[53] that can be used for disinfection include: Scrubbing Bubbles® Multi-Purpose Disinfectant, Fantastik® All-Purpose Cleaner, and Clorox Bleach.

  - BEWARE of "low-splash" bleach - it doesn't disinfect COVID-19!

  - The sick person can clean their own isolation space if they feel up to it.

  - See Chapter 2: Yikes! for many more cleaning tips.

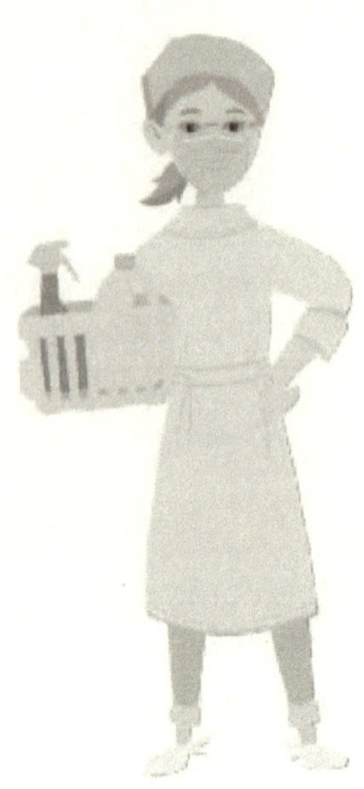

# Keeping Yourself (The Caregiver) Safe

Don't forget to protect yourself and other people around you from getting sick. Wear a mask while with your patient to protect yourself from getting COVID-19, wear a mask around others because you've been exposed to COVID-19, and wear a mask when cleaning so you don't get COVID-19 from surfaces. Yep, that's pretty much all the time! This, paired with washing your hands often with soap and water for at least 20 seconds, will help you protect yourself and others. Review Chapter 2: Yikes! for other ways to keep yourself healthy while providing care for your COVID-19 patient.

**How to use your Personal Protective Equipment:**

* Store PPE in a special location right outside the isolation room and put it on before entering the sick person's room. (PPE includes: mask, kitchen gloves, safety glasses/sunglasses, hat, a protective gown/bathrobe put on backwards, and maybe even plastic bag shoe covers.) You will need at least 2 sets of PPE to use as you cycle through washing your used items.

* Take off PPE immediately after leaving the sick person's room and properly clean or dispose of used items in one of these ways:

- Carefully cover and take items outside to disinfect after you have contact with your patient. Disinfect items while wearing a mask. Leave PPE in direct sunlight for at least 2 hours.

- Wash and dry your PPE in the laundry.

- Bag up what you can't wash and throw it into outside trash containers.

- Wash your hands with soap for at least 20 seconds after putting on AND immediately after taking off your protection. (Get some good lotion for your hands - you'll need it, and you deserve it!)

- Remember not to touch your face while you are cleaning up.

## Your Role As The Caregiver

Your main goal is to support the sick person while staying safe yourself. That's a big job. (**You may be eligible for paid leave; check with your employer.**) Remember that anyone who has been in contact with a known COVID-19 infected person at closer than 6 feet for more than 15 minutes at a time is considered a contact and will have to quarantine for 14 DAYS after exposure! Keep your check-ins short but frequent. Use the phone, FaceTime, and even just talking through the door to communicate regularly with your patient. Read Chapter 4: Oh No! for details on **these caretaking measures**:

- Make sure the patient keeps up with any regular medications they were taking before contracting COVID-19.

- Record any medications taken. Use our symptom tracker in Chapter 8: Track!

- Make sure your patient has lots of fluids to drink. Staying hydrated will help keep any fluids in their lungs loose and easier to cough up.

- Encourage sick individuals to:

  - Stay as active as possible (gently exercise and move, go outside, etc.)

  - Do breathing exercises and change positions (see Chapter 4: Oh

No!)

- Rest as much as needed
- Eat healthy - include their favorite comfort foods!

* Keep a record of the patient's vital signs and symptoms. Turn to Chapter 4: Oh No! for all the details.

  - Get a thermometer to take their temperature.
  - Record their breathing rate (respiration rate): Use a watch/timer to count the number of breaths the patient takes in 30 seconds and multiply that number by 2. (A breath is 1 inhale and 1 exhale.) Do this when they are relaxed, maybe while watching TV.
  - If you have a pulse oximeter, measure the patient's percent oxygen saturation on their second or third finger.

* Monitor your patient for warning signs and worsening symptoms.

  - NOTE - Day 8 of infection is the day of most hospitalizations. Keep a very close eye on your patient's symptoms on days 7-10.
  - This is a big job! If you're worried, seek care earlier rather than waiting. Telehealth (healthcare over the phone/video chat) can be very helpful.

* **Go to the Emergency Room for immediate medical care if your patient:**

  - Has increased or worsening shortness of breath or difficulty breathing
  - Can't say a sentence without taking breaths in between words
  - Has experienced an increase in pain while breathing
  - Develops abdominal pain or chest pain
  - Has an oxygen saturation of 96% or below (95% is the admission threshold in most hospitals)
  - Is confused or acting unlike themself
  - Can't stay awake
  - Has a blue tint to their lips or face
  - Has a new rash, especially on their toes

* Give both regular medicine and symptom-relief medicine to the patient.

* NOTE - Medication may help improve symptoms, or may keep the person's COVID-19 infection from getting worse, but none of these medicines are cures. The only cure is time! **Refer to the medications section in <u>Chapter 4</u>: Oh No! for dosages and details.**

  * Some supplements that can make the infection less severe include:

    - Vitamin D, which can help prevent pneumonia.
    - Zinc, which can help prevent COVID-19 from entering cells.
    - Vitamin C, which can help to prevent and fight COVID-19.[54]

  * Some medications that can lower fever are:

    - Acetaminophen (Tylenol, paracetamol)
    - Alternating doses of ibuprofen (Advil, Motrin)

  * Some medications that can improve cough and congestion are:

    - Guaifenesin (Mucinex, Robitussin)
    - Dextromethorphan (Delsym, Robitussin DM, Nyquil)
    - Pseudoephedrine (Sudafed)

## COVID-19 and Children

We are learning more every day about how kids are affected by COVID-19. At first, it was thought that children don't get this illness. Over time, we have learned that while kids may be less susceptible to COVID-19, they can still catch the virus and can be just as contagious as adults. Most children show few and mild symptoms, but some do become critically ill. All the advice in this handbook applies to kids as well as adults!

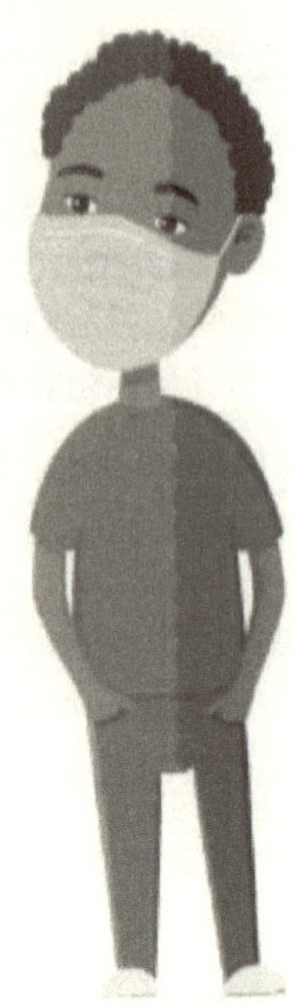

# What should I do if my child has symptoms?[55]

If your child has a fever, cough, or other symptoms of COVID-19, **call** their doctor or nurse. They can tell you what to do and whether your child needs to be seen in person.

If you are taking care of your child at home, the doctor or nurse will tell you what symptoms to watch for. Some children with COVID-19 suddenly get worse after being sick for about a week. The doctor or nurse can tell you when to call the office and when to call for emergency help. For example, you should get emergency help **right away** if your child or baby:

* Has trouble breathing
* Has pain or pressure in their chest
* Has blue lips or face
* Has severe belly pain
* Acts confused or not like themselves
*

Cannot wake up or stay awake

If you have a baby and they are having trouble feeding normally or seem less alert, call your doctor immediately for advice.

Studies have shown that children can have the COVID-19 virus in both their saliva and their feces. One study found a high amount of the COVID-19 virus in the feces and saliva of children who had mild symptoms or were asymptomatic.[56] This may be one reason why kids with COVID-19 are so contagious. Children should be tested for COVID-19 if they show symptoms or come into prolonged contact with someone who has tested positive, just like adults. They need to be isolated if they test positive or are sick.

## Multisystem Inflammatory Syndrome in Children:

Although most kids have a mild form of the illness, there is a risk that any ill child may develop a serious COVID-19-related condition called Multisystem Inflammatory Syndrome in Children (MIS-C[57]). If it is not treated quickly, this inflammation can damage blood vessels and organs throughout a child's body. Careful medical care, hospitalization, and sometimes even the Intensive Care Unit may be needed.

Get your child to the doctor or go to the ER if you notice any of these symptoms:

* Fever lasting more than 24 hours
* Belly pain, vomiting, or diarrhea
* Neck pain
* Rash
* Red or bloodshot eyes
* Redness and/or swelling of the lips, tongue, hands, or feet
* Extra fatigue

Seek emergency care if any of these symptoms worsen, or the child has:

- Inability to wake up/stay awake
- Difficulty breathing
- Chest pain
- New confusion
- A blue tint on the lips or face
- Severe stomach pain

## When To Go Back To "Normal" Life

- **People with COVID-19 who have symptoms** may discontinue isolation under the following conditions.[58]
    - At least 10 days have passed since symptom onset **and**
    - At least 24 hours have passed since resolution of fever without the use of fever-reducing medications **and**
    - Other symptoms have improved.
- **People who have a positive respiratory test for COVID-19 but never developed COVID-19 symptoms** may discontinue isolation when:
    - At least 10 days have passed since the confirmed test **and**
    - NO symptoms have developed.
- Remember that **YOU, the caretaker, need a COVID-19 test** even if you don't have symptoms. As a contact, you need to be in quarantine. Brief interactions are less likely to result in transmission; however, symptoms and the type of interaction (for example, did the infected person cough directly into the face of the exposed individual) remain important.

All household members should be tested for COVID-19 if they were exposed to the COVID-19 patient in the 2-3 days before their symptoms, if any, started.

# Immunity

Nobody knows how long COVID-19 immunity lasts. While the body might develop some protective antibodies after getting COVID-19, it's unknown whether all patients develop this protective response and how long the effect lasts. If you've had COVID-19, you could still get it again. Keep wearing your mask and following daily prevention practices even after you recover! Some people relapse, so keep an eye out for symptoms for several weeks.

Remember to have the sick person in your care get a **flu shot** as soon as it is available and they have recovered from COVID-19. Many COVID-19 symptoms overlap with flu symptoms, so the immunity created by the vaccine will help avoid confusion should they become ill again.

Thank you! You are doing a really important job! You are a COVID HERO and you are keeping many people safe. Take care of yourself, take a break, and stay in touch with family and friends.

In the next chapter, we'll provide information for some other COVID heroes: essential workers. Read on to learn more about how to stay safe and healthy in the workplace.

# WORK! HOW AM I GOING TO HANDLE THIS?

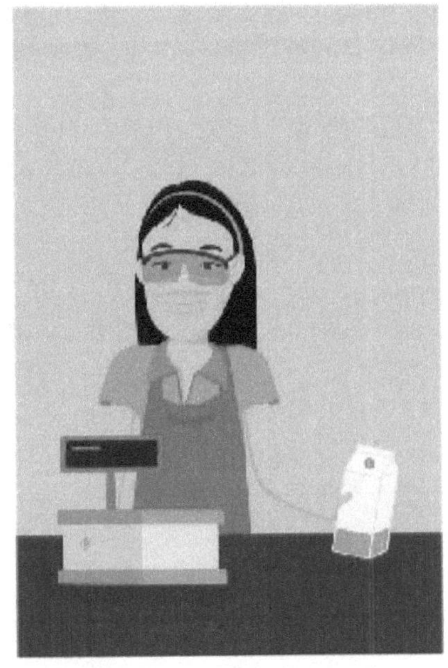

## Chapter 6 Outline

1) What Personal Protective Equipment (PPE) Should You Wear?

    a) Masks

    b) Glasses/Eye Protection

    c) Gloves

2) Prevention While You're Working

    a) Hand Washing

    b) Social Distancing

    c) Worksite Cleaning and Disinfecting

    d) Managing Public Areas

    e) Transportation

    f) Money Handling

    g) Break Rooms

    h) Public Restrooms

    i) After Work

    j) More Tips

3) What to Do If You're an Employer

    a) Employer COVID-19 Health and Safety Plans

    b) Health Checks

    c) Occupation-Specific Health and Safety Guidelines

SO, YOU'VE GOT A REALLY DIFFICULT JOB.

Two, actually: your regular work, and the new job of keeping yourself safe in a COVID-19 world. Luckily, most employers are aware that they share the responsibility of keeping you safe (if you're an employer and want more information, no worries - there's a section below for you!). The CDC wants workers to be protected, too, and they've issued a lot of guidelines to help you stay safe at work (you can check for your specific job's guidelines at the end of this chapter). However, **your safety is ultimately your responsibility**. We've included many practical ways to help you stay safe so you can work, take care of your family, and take care of yourself. Keep an eye out for tips from other sources as they are being updated regularly. This is a great time to share ideas, and we'd love to hear yours.

Details on the best ways to avoid COVID-19 can be found in <u>Chapter 2</u>: Yikes! Use personal protective equipment, keep your hands and the surfaces around you clean, and control your environment by limiting your contact with others.

Sometimes thinking of COVID-19 as big red spiky balls that you have to avoid - as if you were playing a video game - makes it easier to visualize the virus and how to combat it. Limiting your exposure to the virus is the key to staying safe. It doesn't take many virus particles to infect you because they multiply so quickly inside the body.

There's something else that people who work outside the home need to know. Scientists suspect that for every 1 person diagnosed with COVID-19, there may be 10 more who have the virus.[59] Even before they develop symptoms, these people can infect others, like you, who can still get really sick. Coming into contact with many people while you are at work greatly increases your risk of being exposed compared to someone who stays at home. One way you can respond? **Act as if everyone around you has COVID-19**!

Think like a healthcare worker in a COVID-19 ward at the hospital. They have a lower rate of getting COVID-19 than expected because of the enforced use of masks, goggles, handwashing, and protective clothing.

## What Personal Protective Equipment (PPE) Should You Wear?

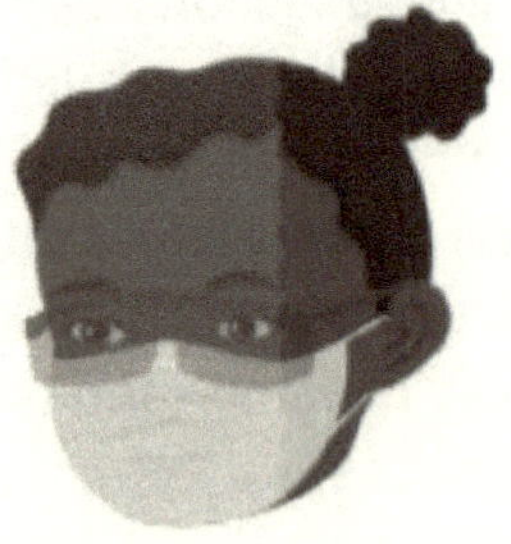

## Masks

**For full information on masks - including types and how to make your own, please read the section on masks in Chapter 2: Yikes!**

**As someone who works around others, you should REALLY have a good mask.**

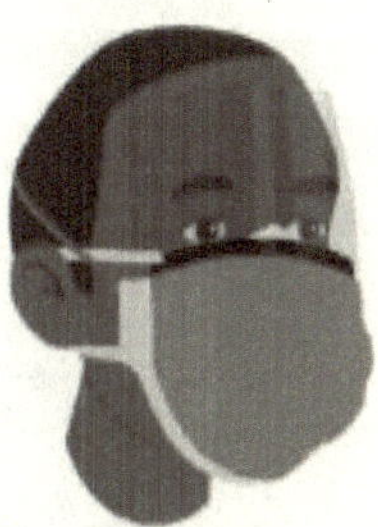

Our nose has 2 sets of cells inside it - goblet and ciliated cells - that are key entry points for the COVID-19 virus. The virus attaches right onto those cells and then multiplies exponentially and travels down into the lungs. This is why it is so important for your mask to cover your mouth AND your nose! And we know it can be a difficult habit to break, but **avoid touching your face** as much as possible, even when wearing a mask. This is a very important way to avoid infection.

Wearing a face mask should NOT impact your ability to breathe and will not cause carbon dioxide overload (surgeons and nurses don't faint from lack of air during long operations!). Air can pass through surgical and cloth masks, while droplets carrying the virus are filtered out. People with respiratory issues should stick to surgical and cloth masks rather than N95 masks, which are thicker and may make breathing difficult for these individuals (N95 masks should be reserved for health workers on the frontline anyway).

NOTE - N95 masks require a special "fit test" to be sized and shaped correctly. Healthcare workers get these fit tests done before working at hospitals - without a fit test, you won't know if your N95 is protecting you!

## How to properly wear your mask:

* Make sure the mask covers your face from the top (bridge) of your nose to under your chin.

* Don't slide the mask up and down on your face - take it off if you don't need to use it.

* Don't touch the front of your mask; COVID-19 viral particles can collect there. Adjust your mask by pulling up on its ear loops.

* **Masks can make you hot, especially when you are moving around. Change your mask if it gets wet, dirty, or sweaty. Keep an extra mask with you at all times while at work.**

* Put on your mask before putting on your gloves (if you need gloves).

* Remove your mask by grabbing the ties - never the front - and pulling it out and away from your face.

* Wash your hands with soap and water for at least 20 seconds before putting your mask on and after removing it.

* Have several cloth masks if possible.

  ‣ Think of your masks as fashion accessories - have fun with them!

'Switch them often (even during your shift) to be sure you are wearing a clean one.

**How to take care of your cloth masks:**

* **Leave them in the sun (for example, on the dash of your car, not hanging from the gear shift) between uses - sunlight breaks down COVID-19 virus.**
* Regularly wash them with soap and water.
* Dry them in the dryer, with a hair dryer, or in the sun.

**Do NOT reuse surgical or N95 masks if they get wet! The filter won't work anymore.**

NOTE - **Masks can affect the lower part of your field of vision**, making it hard to see what's in front of your feet. Make sure to look down when you are navigating stairs, escalators, and cluttered areas.

## Glasses/Eye Protection

Protective glasses are an underused safety item; they can **prevent COVID-19 particles from entering your eyes**. Yes, studies show that COVID-19 transmission can occur through the eyes![60] Most hospitals now require eye protection for employees. It's a good idea for everyone. See Chapter 2: Yikes! for more information.

**To protect your eyes:**

* Don't touch your face and eyes.
* **Wear protective eyewear** (sunglasses, regular glasses, safety glasses, or goggles) along with your mask when at work and out in public.
* Adjust your glasses by moving the arms, not by pushing them up at your nose. Consider eyewear straps to hold them tightly to your head. You can loop your mask into the strap, too, to keep pressure

off your ears.

* **Use a face shield** if your work situation involves possible exposure to sprays and splatters (such as cleaning bars, restaurants, clinics, or bus stations). They are also helpful if you must be very close to other people (like in nail salons, preschools, or home health professions). If shields are not supplied by your employer, they are available online. You can also make your own face shield[61] using a clear 1-liter soda bottle or many other clear plastic materials, like report covers.

  ' Face shields don't replace masks - always wear a mask under your face shield!

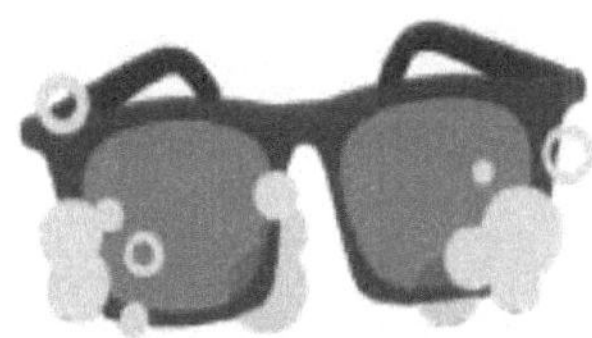

**How to avoid foggy glasses when wearing a mask:**

* Wash your glasses with soapy water, then let them air dry without rinsing (this works, we tried it!).

* Fold a tissue and place it on the bridge of your nose, underneath your glasses.

* Try mild alcohol wipes made for glasses. Let the glasses dry before putting them on so your eyes don't sting.

* If you get a lot of fogging, it means that your mask is not tight enough at the top where your breath is coming out (which means virus particles can get in!). Adjust the straps and the nose piece. **Although filtration works best when your mask fits tightly everywhere, if you need to adjust your mask, it's better to loosen it a bit at the bottom, below your chin, than to make it loose at your nose.**

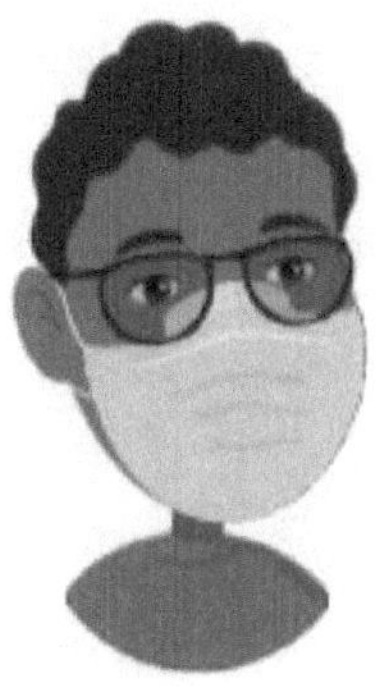

# Gloves

Gloves are a great way to get an extra layer between you and exposed surfaces. See Chapter 2: Yikes! for full information on medical-style gloves, cloth gloves, kitchen gloves, and the best ways to use them.

## Prevention While You're Working

## Hand Washing

**Wash** your hands for 20 seconds or use hand sanitizer for 20 seconds. The CDC has published these occupational guidelines on handwashing:[62]

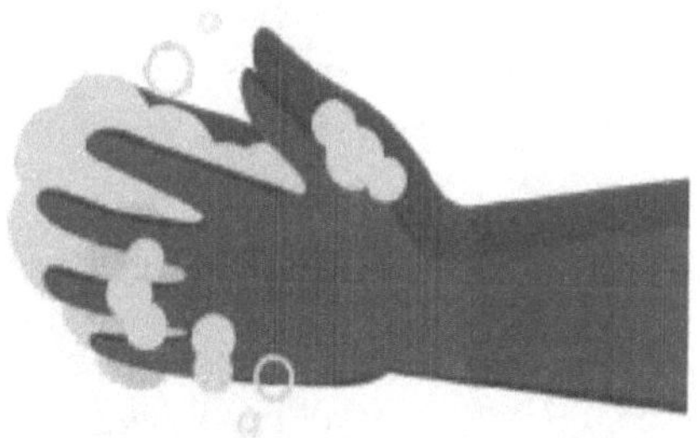

* Key times to clean hands include:
    * Before, during, and after preparing food
    * Before eating food
    * After using the restroom
    * After blowing your nose, coughing, or sneezing

* Additional times to clean hands on the job include:
    * Before and after work shifts
    * Before and after work breaks
    * After touching frequently touched surfaces
    * After interacting with customers who are visibly ill
    * After putting on, touching, or removing cloth face coverings
    * After touching objects that have been handled by customers, such as utensils, menus, cups, or trash
    * After touching dirty surfaces like floors, walls, soiled carriers, and equipment

**Even if you wear gloves** for these activities, **wash your hands** often. Gloves get dirty on the inside, too.

**Tips from One Good Turn:**

* Keep hand sanitizer with you for any time you can't wash your hands right away.

* **Carry your own soap, just like you do hand sanitizer**: Cut up a bar of soap (which is cheaper than liquid soap) and toss a piece in a bag; carry it and a small towel in a protected bag that only you use. Now you can easily wash your face as well as your hands. Wash the towel every day.

* Keep some thick **hand lotion** with you, too - hands can get really chapped with frequent washing!

* Use gloves, especially if your work involves cleaning surfaces or touching people or items used by multiple people. Reusable cloth gloves are fine if washed regularly and are much more comfortable than plastic or rubber gloves. Remember not to touch your face with your gloved hands.

* **Wash your gloved hands! You can even use hand sanitizer on gloves.** This is another way to protect your skin from cleaning

products and the virus.

## Social Distancing

Stay 6 feet (72 inches) away from everyone.

- Your wingspan (the distance from middle fingertips when both arms are outstretched) is usually about the same as your height - use your wingspan to help estimate a 6-foot distance.
- Measure 6 feet away from where you stand at work and mark a safe spot for others.
- You can also use a standard piece of notebook paper (which is 8.5 x 11 inches) - 7 paper-lengths is a good distance.

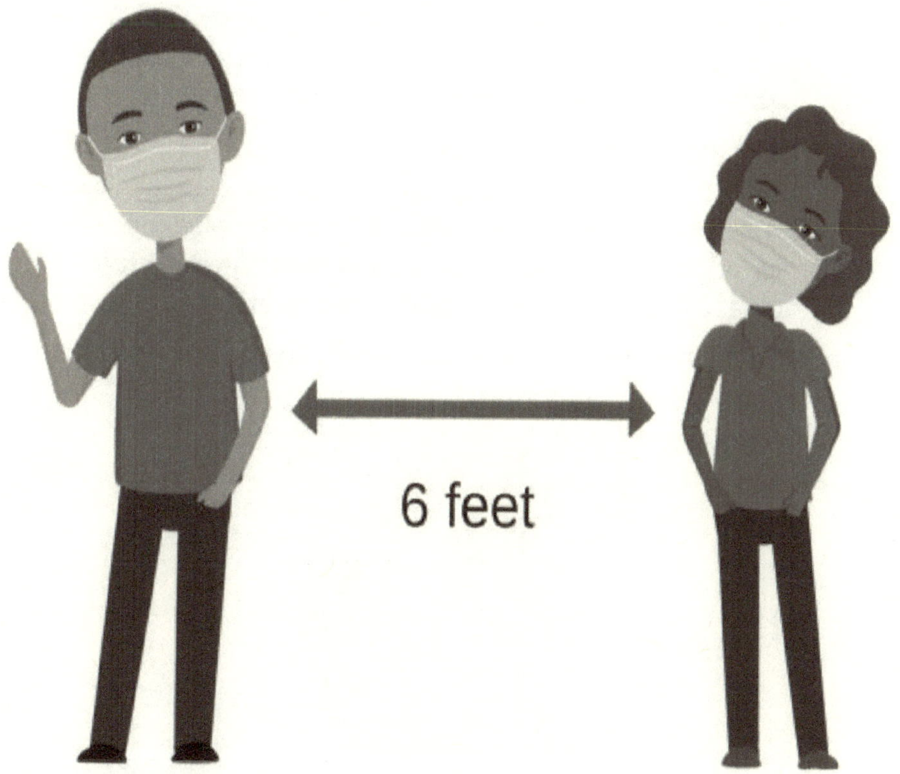


Use a protective barrier.

* If distance is not in your control, you can put a protective barrier, like a window or plexiglass (often called a sneeze guard) between yourself and customers.

* If you work at a register without protection, try using clear plastic to make your own shield. Trim and hang up a clear shower curtain. You could also wear a face shield!

* Remember to wash/change out your protective barrier (while wearing gloves) at the beginning of every day or shift.

If you must work in a crowd:

* Know and follow your state/local guidelines on the number or percent occupancy a room can have at one time - **you may be the one to notice that there are too many people gathered**. Ask your boss or company to make and post a written policy so employees can safely protect themselves and the business from fines and closure.

* Background music and lots of people means that speaking volume increases, and, along with it, viral particles and droplets are projected stronger and further. **Consider lowering the music volume to enable people to speak more quietly.**

* Clean often, while wearing protection. Consider using a face shield over your mask while at work.

## Worksite Cleaning and Disinfecting

Remember to routinely clean and disinfect frequently touched surfaces, such as workstations, cash registers, touch screens, door handles, tables, and countertops. Also disinfect reusable items between uses. It is best to **let the product stay on the surface for at least 1 minute before wiping it clean.**[63] It takes 1-5 minutes for bleach to fully destroy the virus by breaking down its cell walls. Here are some cleaning options:

* Correctly **diluted household bleach**:
  * Prepare a bleach solution by mixing: 5 tablespoons (⅓cup) bleach per gallon of room temperature water or 4 teaspoons bleach per quart of room temperature water
* Bleach wipes
* EPA-approved cleaners
  * Scrubbing Bubbles® Multi-Purpose Disinfectant
  * Fantastik® All-Purpose Cleaner
  * Clorox Bleach (Click here for more[64])
  * Lysol Disinfectant Spray
  * Lysol Disinfectant Max Cover Mist
  * Always wear gloves - bleach and cleaning supplies are rough on skin.

## Managing Public Areas

Okay, this is almost like a real-life video game: **Can you get to work and back without touching anything - including your face?** Bonus points for not getting stuck in a crowd of people! Public transportation and other public spaces are high-risk areas since car door handles, door knobs, crosswalk buttons, and other frequently touched surfaces can harbor COVID-19 viral particles. Here are some additional tips:

* Maintain a 6-foot zone around you whenever possible.
* Mask up!

* Wear 1 glove while running errands/commuting - use the gloved hand to open doors or press buttons and your other hand for personal items, like reaching into your purse or backpack for your keys and wallet.
* If you must touch commonly used surfaces (such as door handles, stair railings, or subway grab bars) place a barrier between your hand and the object, like a tissue, gloves, or a plastic grocery bag. Even your sleeves are better than nothing!
* Open doors with your foot or back.
* Take the stairs. Try not to touch handrails unless balance is an issue. If you need support, wear gloves.
* Avoid elevators; mask up and ride alone if possible.
* If you get too close to someone or encounter a cough or sneeze, stop breathing for a few counts. Exhale first when you breathe again.
* Pay attention to ventilation so that you don't stand or sit downwind of crowds.
* If possible, stay in well-ventilated, sunny places, near open doors.

## Transportation

* When riding in a car with others, keep the windows down, even if you need AC (you'd be using the AC anyway!). Keep music soft to avoid speaking loudly.
* For Uber/rideshare, public transit, and air travel tips, see the section on travel in Chapter 2: Yikes!

## Money Handling

* Consider wearing gloves when handling money.
* Place money in a tray on the counter, not into your customer's hands.
* Try touchless pay methods like Apple Pay or debit/credit cards that have the customer do the work.

* Keep a bottle of hand sanitizer on the counter for you and others to use.

## Break Rooms

**Break rooms are one of the riskiest areas for COVID-19 transmission.**

* Use disposable plates, utensils, and cups.
* Be careful when sitting at tables; clean them as you do customer areas. If you must, it is alright to sit at the same table as others, but sit 6 feet apart and staggered (not directly across from each other).
* Pay attention to ventilation - look for the airflow vents and don't sit downwind of any groups of people eating since their masks will be off.
* Instead, eat and take your breaks outside. Control your environment! Stay away from people without masks (for example, people who are eating, drinking, or smoking).
* Try to bring foods that don't need to be microwaved. Microwaves are hotspots for crowds and frequently touched surfaces.

## Public Restrooms

**Restrooms are another very high-risk area for COVID-19 transmission.** Surfaces are dirty, ventilation is poor, and restrooms are used by many people for a wide range of reasons. COVID-19 has been found in feces, so be careful when you flush. A "toilet plume," can happen when the force of the toilet flush sprays virus particles (and other particles) into the air. Close the lid BEFORE flushing or, if there is no lid, hold your breath and step away quickly!

Remember to wash your hands after using the toilet. Avoid hand dryers as they can spread COVID-19 on surfaces into the air. Don't linger in public restrooms.

## After Work

To help lower the chance of bringing COVID-19 into your home, change out of your work clothes as soon as you enter your home.

- Take off and leave your shoes outside the door.
- Immediately wash your face or take a shower.
- Remove potentially exposed clothing and immediately put it into a designated laundry bag.
- Avoid the kitchen and living areas until you've cleaned up.
- Have comfortable clothing and slippers to wear only at home.
- Laundry: It is safe to wash potentially contaminated clothes in a machine. Drying your clothes in a dryer helps to kill any remaining virus particles. Be sure to wear a mask while laundering your work clothing.

## More tips

**Things you can do to stay healthy:** Check out suggestions for vitamin supplements, breathing exercises, health conditions, and more in Chapter 2: Yikes!

**If you do get sick, stay home and get tested**: You may be able to do this through your work site - many health departments also now have free testing.

**If you care for others:** Many employers can offer you paid leave if you must stay home to care for yourself or someone else with COVID-19. Check your options (your employer may get to take your paid leave as a direct tax break!).

Remember to get a **flu shot** as soon as it is available - many COVID-19 symptoms overlap with flu symptoms, so the immunity given by the vaccine will help prevent confusion should you become ill.

# What To Do If You're An Employer

As noted by the CDC[65] and OSHA,[66] as an employer, you should have a COVID-19 health and safety plan to protect and share with all employees. Involve your staff while developing protocols - you can use this chapter's practical suggestions to protect yourself and your staff.

## Employer COVID-19 Health and Safety Plans

* Provide work-appropriate personal protective equipment (PPE) for your staff.

* Take steps to help prevent the spread of COVID-19 if an employee is sick.[67] Actively encourage sick employees to stay home. Sick employees should NOT return to work until the criteria[68] to discontinue home isolation are met, in consultation with healthcare providers and state and local health departments.

* Provide information on who to contact if employees become sick.

* Implement flexible sick leave and other supportive policies and practices. Follow the laws that provide emergency sick leave[69] for family caretakers.

* Institute measures to physically separate and increase distance between employees and customers:

  * Place signs throughout the store to remind employees and customers to stay 6 feet apart and to wear masks covering both their nose and mouth. The CDC has many infographics available for printing.[70]

  * Move the electronic payment terminal further from the cash register.

  * Create visual cues, such as floor decals, colored tape, or signs, to indicate where customers should stand during check out.

  * Add a barrier (sneeze guard) between employees and customers.

* Designate a staff person to be responsible for responding to any COVID-19 concerns and reporting them to you. Employees should know who this person is and how to contact them.

* Provide employees with accurate information about COVID-19, how

it spreads, and the risks of exposure while at work.

* Provide training on proper handwashing[71] techniques and other routine infection-control precautions. This will help prevent the spread of many diseases, including COVID-19.

* Provide employees with access to soap, clean running water, and drying materials, or alcohol-based hand sanitizers containing at least 60% alcohol at their worksite.

* Provide disposable disinfectant wipes so that employees can wipe down commonly touched work surfaces, such as workstations, cash registers, door handles and knobs, countertops, and self-service refrigerator/freezer doors and handles. For disinfection, use products that meet the EPA's criteria[72] for use against COVID-19. Follow instructions on the label to ensure safe and effective use of the product.

* For food-contact surfaces, follow cleaning and sanitization practices according to the FDA 2017 Food Code.[73]

* Provide tissues and no-touch disposal containers for employees.

* Conduct frequent cleaning and disinfection of employee break rooms, rest areas, and other common areas. Make sure plenty of paper towels are available. Spread tables and chairs as far apart as possible.

* Encourage employees to bring food that does not need microwaving. Kitchens and other common areas are hotspots for crowds.

* Create outside break areas.

* Place posters that encourage staying home when sick, covering coughs and sneezes, and frequent handwashing at the entrance to your workplace and in other areas where they will be seen. Restrooms are great places to put handwashing posters.

* And of course, follow all applicable local, state, and federal regulations and public health agency guidelines.

# Health Checks

Employers may institute daily health checks of employees before they enter the facility. The goal is to keep sick employees home and therefore avoid spreading the virus. Examples of checks include taking temperatures with a laser/forehead scan, issuing a symptom questionnaire, or responding to screening questions on a mobile app.

NOTE - these apps must be HIPAA compliant; health information should be protected so that it cannot be used against individuals and, if given to a third party, will not contain any identifying information.

# Occupation-Specific Health and Safety Guidelines

Visit the CDC website for occupation-specific guidelines.

**Airlines and Airports**

    Aircraft Maintenance Workers

**Delivery and Ground Transportation**

    Airline Catering Kitchen Workers
    Airline Catering Truck Drivers
    Airline Customer Service and Gate Agents
    Airport Baggage and Cargo Handlers
    Airport Custodial Staff
    Airport Passenger Assistance Workers
    Airport Retail or Food Service Workers
    Food and Grocery Pick-up and Delivery Drivers
    Long-Haul Truck Drivers
    Mail and Parcel Delivery Drivers

**Shipping**

    Maritime Pilots

**Public Transportation**

    Bus Transit Operators
    Rail Transit Operators

    Rideshare, Taxi, Limo, and Other Passenger Drivers
    Transit Maintenance Workers
    Transit Station Workers

## Personal Services
    Bank employees
    Bank employers
    Nail Salon Employees
    Nail Salon Employers

## Food Services
    Agricultural Workers and Employers
    Grocery and Food Retail Workers
    Meat and Poultry Processors
    School Nutrition Professionals and Volunteers
    Seafood Processing Workers

## Manufacturing and Industrial
    Construction Workers
    Manufacturing Workers and Employers
    Miners

## Public Services and Sanitation
    Fire Fighters and EMS Providers
    Law Enforcement Officers
    Sanitation and Wastewater Workers
    Waste Collectors and Recycler

It may feel like the entire world has been put on pause, but life goes on, and the workforce must adapt to our "new normal." Keep these recommendations on hand and reference them (in addition to the CDC and OSHA, of course!) as needed.

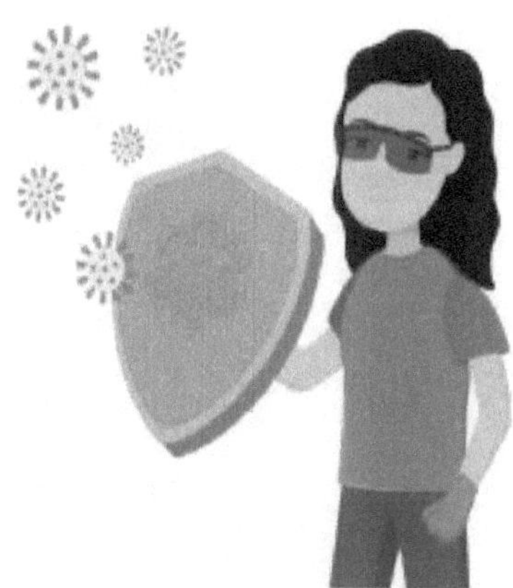

Work isn't the only place where adapting to COVID can be difficult. In the next chapter, we'll provide information about how to handle returning to school while keeping children, teachers, and staff healthy. Keep in mind that the CDC is still solidifying guidelines for returning to school - always check CDC.gov for the most up-to-date information.

# SCHOOL! HOW DO I LEARN SAFELY?

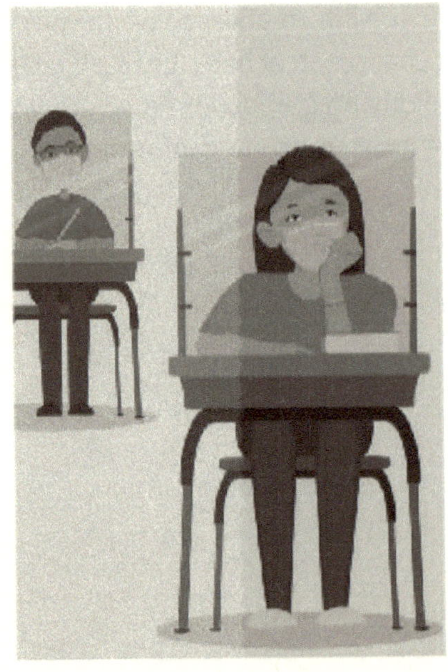

## Chapter 7 Outline

1) Part 1 - School Strategies For Reopening

    a) Dual Online/In-Person Options

    b) Alternating Days, Weeks, or Start Times

    c) Cohort or "Pandemic Pod" Strategy

d) Students with Disabilities/Special Needs

2) Part 2 - For Teachers and School Staff

   a) Back to School Basics

      i) Social Distancing in the Classroom

      ii) Ventilation and Sunlight

      iii) Cleaning

      iv) Food

      v) Restrooms

      vi) Homework and Schoolwork

      vii) Elective Classes and Activities

      viii) Take Care of Yourself

   b) Elementary School

   c) Middle and High School

   d) University

3) Part 3 - For Parents/Guardians and Students

   a) Back to School Basics

      i) Getting Ready

      ii) Food

      iii) Restrooms

      iv) Buses and Carpooling

   b) Elementary School Parents/Guardians

   c) Middle and High School Students

   d) University Students

      i) Housing

      ii) Food

      iii) Prepare Before You Get Sick

The question of whether and how to reopen schools is one of the most complicated and important challenges of the pandemic. We at One Good Turn do not advocate that schools reopen or stay closed. Those decisions are best left in the hands of leaders and individual families who can appropriately assess the many risks and benefits of returning to school within each school district and community. However, **just as we do in our global healthcare work, One Good Turn can offer practical ideas to best protect those at risk of infection in the imperfect environments where they must live and work.** In the spirit of teamwork and protection for the dedicated families and professionals who are responsible for advancing the education of young people everywhere, we offer the information in this chapter as suggestions for those who must attend and work at schools. We hope they will provide a helpful framework for individuals to make their own best plans and choices. Please read Chapter 6: Work! for more information for teachers and students.

Teachers and education professionals have an invaluable role in educating today's children. COVID-19 has brought new challenges to this school year, and we at One Good Turn recognize and appreciate your service. Thank you to teachers everywhere for your dedication to learning and your service to society.

# Part 1 - School Strategies for Reopening

There are three basic strategies for reopening schools. Your school will probably do something like one of these. Here are some things to note about each.

## Dual Online/In-Person Options

Many schools are planning both online and in-person options for classes. Teachers should seek out support to manage both in-person and online student groups.

If you (the student) must choose between either online or in-person classes for the whole semester, consider:

* Do you have medical conditions that put you at high-risk of getting severe illness from COVID-19?
* Does someone you live with have a medical condition that puts

them at high-risk if they get COVID-19?

* Do you have easy access to online communication?

* Does your living and travel situation present challenges to staying safe during the pandemic?

* Do your learning strengths or living conditions make in-person school a better way for you to learn?

* In some cases, online classes may affect your degree plan. Will an online option affect your graduation date?

**NOTE - Be aware that school districts who do not receive responses from parents/guardians on schooling arrangements may assume that in-person schooling is the default choice of the family.**

If you (the student) can choose to attend either an online or an in-person class at any time throughout the semester, consider:

* Are you feeling ill?

* Is someone you interacted with for more than 15 minutes feeling ill?

* Are you putting yourself at risk by going to school or by staying home?

## Alternating Days, Weeks, or Start Times

Some schools will have half of a class attend for one part of the week and the other half attend for the other part of the week (students not attending in person will have online instruction). Schools may also have students arrive at different times to prevent crowding. For this method to be effective, everyone involved should practice proper COVID-19 prevention habits, **especially teachers and staff**.

## Cohort or "Pandemic Pod" Strategy

This strategy has groups of students (such as elementary school classes or smaller groups) interact with each other only. This strategy is an option if small groups of students wish to get together in person for online school or to homeschool. For this strategy to be effective, it is important that the cohort limits all interactions with other people (including other cohorts, teachers, or friends). If you or your child's school decide to implement this strategy, be sure you know who is in your child's cohort and do your best to adhere to the expectations (for example, don't arrange playdates with anyone outside of the cohort!).

## Students with Disabilities/Special Needs

The CDC recommends that students with disabilities/special needs be allowed to attend school, if possible, and recommends that these students be taught in a cohort group (as described above) due to the increased risk of serious complications with infection. This strategy can help minimize their risk of exposure to an infectious person. For more information see the CDC's recommendations.[74]

# Part 2 - For Teachers and School Staff

## Back to School Basics

Teachers, school administrators, custodians, nursing and counseling staff, cafeteria workers, librarians, bus drivers, coaches - every professional in the academic world will be profoundly affected by COVID-19. One Good Turn recognizes that we cannot anticipate or advise you on every aspect of your work life. You are the expert in your field.

School, no matter how it reopens, will not look the way it did back in the "olden days" of last fall. New burdens around safety and sanitation will be added to the tremendous challenges of adapting academic goals and teaching capabilities to online and in-person settings.

Guidelines for schools change often. If you're not sure what your state's policies are, you can look for them here.[75] Local school district policies will directly affect your school. Stay up to date on all communications from district and school administrators.

**Encourage your students to stay home if they are sick** - this is a crucial step to keep COVID-19 from getting into schools! Work with your students so they know they can miss school without repercussions. Ask your students (or their parents/guardians) to check their temperature each morning before school. If they are running a fever [oral/skin temperature greater than 100.4°F (38°C)] or have a cough or other symptoms of COVID-19, they should stay home. If the student has an immediate family member or another close contact with COVID-19 they should stay home. As a teacher or staff member, it is very important that you also stay home if you are sick, as you probably interact with more people daily than your students do!

You may go through a daily **check-in station.** Your school should have a way to **screen each person entering the building for COVID-19 symptoms**. Usually this involves a forehead temperature check and screening questions about known exposure to and prior testing for COVID-19. It is best to set up a designated check-in station outside the school building that anyone entering the school must go through each day. Keep in mind that if a person has an elevated skin temperature, it could be from hot weather or physical exertion, so the temperature check should be repeated after the person has rested indoors. If still elevated, then the reading should be confirmed with an oral temperature. To limit exposure, parents/guardians, friends, and family should not come inside school - use a designated drop off area and one-way entrance system.

Volunteers help run check-in stations so that the teachers can attend to their students. These volunteers can also help with the ongoing disinfection processes in school. Limit the number of volunteers present at any time and require that volunteers participate in screening and temperature checks.

Inside your school, plan a one-way route through the school, including stairways, to avoid face-to-face passing for teachers and students.

**Students who get sick at school should be given a mask and placed in isolation**. Have a comfortable space planned in advance for sick students to wait in while transportation home is arranged. Wearing a mask and gloves, put the student's belongings in a plastic bag and give them to the student or parent/guardian. Wash your hands after handling those items and disinfect the student's desk and chair, common classroom areas, and frequently touched surfaces as soon as possible.

**If you are told that one of your students tests positive for COVID-19**, contact your principal, school medical staff, or administration. **The school administration, not the teacher, must notify the student's direct contacts while protecting the student's anonymity.** Know your school's protocol, as you will get lots of questions about it. Depending on the timing of the positive test, you may need to evacuate the classroom, open outside doors and windows, turn on fans, and clean the student's desk. You should then wait at least 24 hours before disinfecting all common areas and frequently touched surfaces in the classroom and opening it up for reuse.[76]

**Use personal protective equipment (PPE). Wear a mask at all times** and consider wearing a face shield if you'll be in close proximity with others. Remember to wash/sanitize your hands after physical contact occurs - aim for no contact, although that may be unrealistic. Gloves (cloth are fine) can help keep your hands clean and away from your face and students' germs. See Chapter 2: Yikes! for more on good PPE usage. Don't touch your face and encourage your students not to touch theirs. Consider using a face mask with a clear visible expression panel (available online) so students can see more of your face as you teach.

Children will also be getting used to using PPE. Just as you are a role model for so many other important behaviors, you will be a model for PPE usage. Normalize germ-aware behaviors for your students and set a positive example, as these habits are now a part of our daily lives.

### Social Distancing in the Classroom

COVID-19 is most easily transmitted when many people are indoors in close proximity. Social distancing, combined with PPE, is the best way to prevent spread. Social distancing will look different for every classroom and activity. Plan activities and class orientations that keep students away from each other and from you. "Close contact" is more than 15 minutes at less than 6 feet; **set a timer during your one-on-one and small group activities**.

Try to **arrange desks to be at least 6 feet apart** and facing in the same direction. If using tables, seat students on only one side of the table and mark the floor to keep chairs spaced apart. Use sneeze guards or partitions, especially if desks cannot be placed 6 feet apart (test dividing folders are a good temporary substitute for sneeze guards). Mark 6 feet of space with decals on the floor in other areas of the room and hallways as well.

COVID-19 particles are proven to spread further when a person speaks or sings loudly. Is a microphone and speaker system available? See if your district or school will provide one. This will allow your students to hear you better so you can avoid raising your voice as you speak through your mask.

**Ventilation and Sunlight**

Take a good look at the ventilation system in your classroom. Does air flow in a specific direction due to vent placement? If so, **avoid seating arrangements where linear airflow could create a path of viral spread from one student to others**. Increasing general circulation from added fans or ceiling fans is helpful. Open windows, classroom doors, and outside doors if possible. Keep window shades up to let direct sunlight into your classroom as sunlight is proven to deactivate COVID-19 particles. After cleaning, leave items that must be shared on windowsills in the sun for as long as possible between uses. Although it will be challenging, try teaching a class outside if the weather is good! In addition to making it easier for your students to spread out, sunlight breaks down COVID-19 virus particles and makes vitamin D.[77]

## Cleaning

Cleaning and disinfection will quickly become a routine part of your day! Set up a schedule with your students to wipe down all desks and chairs regularly (for example, at the end of lunch break, at the beginning and end of the day, or before a new student uses the desk). Wipe down all frequently used hard surfaces, such as computers, handrails, and door handles more often. NOTE - Hard and soft surfaces have different rules; look here[78] for more information. Ask that your administration designate a person to clean common areas during the day, such as a staff member or a parent/guardian volunteer cleaner.

Don't let children share items (like books, pencils, or crayons). If possible, make sure each student has their own materials and disinfect or wash items between each use. See the CDC's guidelines for disinfection[79] for more details. Get your students involved in managing their environment by asking them to help you with cleaning routines. Pedals and other options make it easier for students to open doors and trash cans with their feet.

If sinks are available in classrooms or hallways, keep them stocked with soap. Bar soap is fine. Hand sanitizer stations should be placed at all classroom and gathering area doorways. If your school cannot do this, give a squirt of hand sanitizer to your students before they enter the classroom.

## Food

It is safest to bring your food from home. Bring your own full water bottle/drink and encourage your students to bring water bottles also, to avoid drinking fountains. Both students and teachers should eat more than 6 feet away from other people. Eat outside whenever possible! If eating inside, you can use paper towels as placemats for each student.

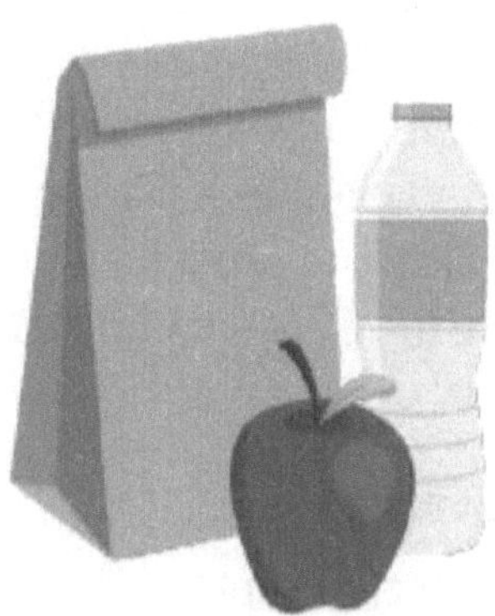

If possible, snacks and lunches distributed to students should be pre-packaged or individually served by a designated person in PPE (especially masks and gloves). Snacks and rewards can also be put in student trays or on desks when students are out of the classroom.

Cafeterias will need the same distancing/cleaning/ventilation/hand sanitizing as the classroom but with even more diligence since students will have to take their masks off to eat. Loud voices can also increase viral spread. Look for ways to give your students a needed break that won't increase indoor noise - perhaps extra recess time outside, or permission for all to use headphones, or a fun movie to watch during lunch.

## Restrooms

Restrooms are one of the most high-risk areas for COVID-19 transmission! Don't spend extra time in the stalls. Look at our restroom section in Chapter 6: Work! for more details on the safest ways to use public restrooms. Limit how many of your students are in the restroom at a time. Use foot pedals for flushing (with signs so no one accidentally touches the flush handle). Pedals and other options make it easier for students to open doors and trash cans with their feet. Ventilate the restroom as much as possible, don't line up students near the door, ensure that soap dispensers always have soap, and provide paper towels instead of air dryers. Give a squirt of hand sanitizer to your students before they reenter the classroom.

## Homework and Schoolwork

Have students complete and turn in assignments digitally. Otherwise, set up assignment turn-in trays and individual mailboxes so you don't handle paperwork directly. Make sure your students walk up to the trays or mailboxes one at a time. Put worksheets or assignments on their desk when students are not in class. Use paper handouts instead of shared books and try to make sure there are enough materials (scissors, colored pencils, rulers) for individual use.

## Elective Classes and Activities

Sports, PE, music, art, and special events all pose different challenges. A good practice is to move as few people around the school community as possible, which means non-core class ("specials") teachers may come to individual classrooms while students stay in one place. PPE and cleaning routines are even more important for teachers who move between classrooms, both for self-protection and to avoid unintentionally spreading the virus. It's a big responsibility.

PE classes and sports leagues should find activities that allow students to stay 6 feet apart. High-exertion activities indoors can easily spread viruses - many super-spread events have occurred during high intensity exercise classes.[80] Plan moderate activities, such as stretching or yoga. Cardio activities can be done outside if there is plenty of space. Students may find that breathing heavily through a mask feels difficult. Give students time and space to adjust masks and catch their breath. Note that dry masks do not cause oxygen deficiency, but wet, sweaty masks will be ineffective and harder to breathe through.[81]

Band and choir classes will have to plan for the documented increase in the amount of air droplets produced when singing and blowing on instruments.[82] Music students can practice alone or focus on music reading and listening skills.

School dances or field trips have many unknown opportunities for exposure. Pick virtual events (like virtual tours or school-spirit events) instead. Make sure you know about any online or alternative learning options your school or district may have and share these options with your students.

**Take Care of Yourself**

Finally, please make sure to **take care of yourself**. As a teacher or staff member, you will interact with many more people than your students do (especially if your school is using an alternate days or weeks strategy). Keep yourself healthy and COVID-19 free! **When you get home from school**:

1. Take off your shoes outside the door (leave them in the sun if you c

2. Wipe down your backpack, lunch box, and purse

3. Remove potentially exposed clothing and put it in a laundry bag

4. Wash your hands and face with soap and water, or take a shower

5. Change into comfortable, at-home-only clothes

6. Get some exercise, relax, do a few of your favorite activities - take a

See Chapter 2: Yikes! for more details on COVID-19 safety practices. See Chapter 4: Work! for more ideas about the workplace.

**Tip:** Get your annual **flu shot** as soon as possible once it is available in the fall. Many COVID-19 symptoms overlap with flu symptoms, so the immunity created by the vaccine will help avoid confusion should you become ill.

As an academic professional, you will be responsible for a new frontier of learning and communication during this pandemic. Below are some **grade-specific considerations**.

# Elementary School

Parents/guardians may need reassurance that it's okay to tell you if their child feels sick, uncomfortable, or stressed. Be in contact frequently. Try to send out regular class reports that include updates from your school's health officer.

Talk to your students regularly about COVID-19 safety. Teach an "About COVID-19" lesson plan on the first days of school. Portray COVID-19 illness prevention as a team effort and explain to your students that they are keeping themselves and others safe. Younger students may be used to hugs or high fives. Give lots of smiles instead. Create a fun project for the classroom where students come up with a few distanced ways they can greet one another, such as a dance, a song, or hand signals. Ask parents to help you reinforce the habits you teach in the classroom by supporting and encouraging them at home as well.

## Middle and High School

Students in this age group may go to multiple classrooms with different students each day, so one person with COVID-19 can spread the virus very quickly. If possible, stagger passing periods, create a one-way traffic flow through your school, and have students go directly to their classrooms when they get to school instead of waiting in a common area. Encourage your students to eat lunch outside or in classrooms. If your school allows, let your students go home or leave campus for lunch.

Share clear guidelines with your students about options made for COVID-19, including possible online assignments and which in-school activities they can adapt if they are uncomfortable. Make sure your students know what options they have if they need to take care of a sick family member (see Chapter 5: Help! for more resources). Maintain a welcoming and open attitude - the goal is to keep students in school. Dropout rates are higher for those with extended absences and students above age 16. Anticipate tutoring and special learning needs for students who have extenuating circumstances. Keep school wifi available after hours; many students and families do homework in the school parking lot.

Finally, watch for COVID-19 bullying. This could include behavior such as attempting to infect classmates with COVID-19, stigmatizing a student who has COVID-19, or making fun of students who might be at high risk of COVID-19 infection due to obesity, race, or health conditions. Lead by example and show your students how to keep an open mind and provide a non-judgemental atmosphere for everyone at the school. Listen to your students and provide them with the support they need.

## University

Options for online learning are greater at the college level. University professors and their students will become leaders in digital learning. Develop clear guidelines for your students - and yourself - about exceptions you are willing to make due to COVID-19. Can students opt to do assignments online? Which in-school activities can be accomplished with minimal risk? How can small class gatherings be safe and productive for all? Make sure your students know what options they have if they need to take care of a sick family member (see Chapter 5: Help! for more resources).

## Part 3 - For Parents/Guardians and Students

School, no matter how it reopens, will not look the way it did back in the "olden days" of last fall. New burdens around safety and sanitation will be added to the tremendous challenges of adapting academic goals and teaching capabilities to online and in-person settings. Let's explore ways to keep everybody healthy at school during this pandemic.

## Back to School Basics for Parents/Guardians and Students

Strategies to fight COVID-19 are most effective when everyone participates! Look for communications from your school district and be aware of your state's policies. If you're not sure what your state's policies are, you can look for them here.[83]

By now you know the best ways to protect yourself from COVID-19:

- Be prepared
- Stay home if you are sick
- Wear a mask
- Keep your distance from others
- Keep your hands, face, and belongings clean

Here are some basic tips for school and where to find more information about each topic in this handbook.

**Getting ready**

Make yourself a COVID-19 kit: a few masks, a small bottle of hand sanitizer, some disinfectant wipes, a small piece of soap, some gloves (cloth are fine), lotion, chapstick, and even sunscreen (since it will be wiped off with your mask). Add a pair of sunglasses for eye protection and you'll be ready for anything. Keep your stuff in a bag that you can toss into whatever you carry with you.

**Parents, take your child's temperature daily** before school (and anytime they feel ill!). Make preparations in advance with your family, friends, work, or coworkers so you can keep your child home if they aren't feeling well (see Chapter 4: Oh No! for a list of symptoms). It is important that all students, regardless of age, **stay home if they are sick** - this keeps COVID-19 from getting into schools in the first place! Check your child's temperature each morning before going to school. If they are running a fever [oral/skin temperature greater than 100.4°F [38°C]], they should stay home.

**Wear a mask at all times** when outside of the home. See Chapter 2: Yikes! for details on mask fit and efficacy and much more PPE info.

Parents, let your student choose their mask. Offer comfortable 3-layered masks with designs and colors they prefer; it will make the mask easier to wear all day. Once you find a style that works, buy several so they can be used in rotation throughout the day and laundered often. Have your child practice wearing a mask at home for extended periods so that they are used to wearing a mask all day before heading to school.

Keep your distance (see Chapter 6: Work!). **Teach your children what 6 feet of space looks like** so they can get used to social distancing before school starts. Give them a 6-foot measuring tape or string. Stress the importance of staying on floor markings for when standing in lines.

Develop good hand washing habits (see Chapter 2: Yikes! For more details). Parents, teach your children to to correctly wash their hands **for 20 seconds** and to use hand sanitizer for 20 seconds. **Show your kids how to wash under their fingernails!** Instruct them to do this after coughing, touching their face, using the restroom, touching door handles and stair rails, and before and after touching commonly used items. Come up with a 20 second song, poem, or saying to recite while washing their hands that they can easily remember. Give kids a small bottle of hand sanitizer they can keep with them.

Students should **create a routine** when they get home to:

1. Take off shoes outside the door (leave them in the sun if you can!)

2. Wipe down backpacks, lunch boxes, and/or binders

3. Wash hands and face with soap and water

4. Bathe or shower

5. Change into clothes just for home

6. Place potentially exposed clothing, including cloth masks, into a lau bag

7. Take a break, get outside, or play some music. Try some non-electro activities - make de-stressing a priority for all!

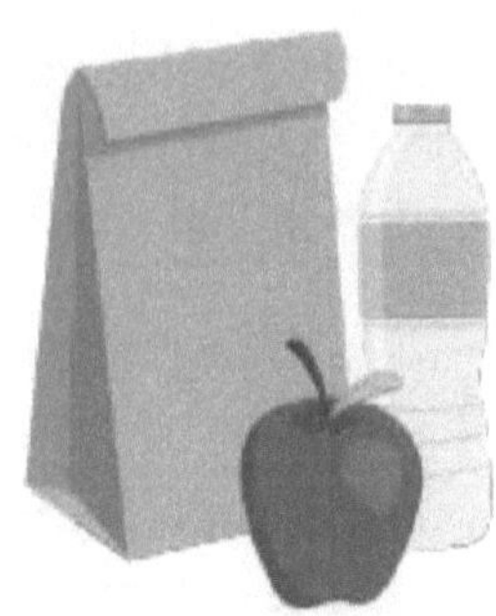

### Food

It is best to bring lunch, drinks, and snacks, and water bottles from home to minimize the need to stand in line and eat food prepared by others. Try disposable eating utensils, plates, and cups, or keep closeable containers in your lunch bag to wash at home. Add disinfecting wipes to your lunch bag. Wash/sanitize your hands before and after eating.

### Restrooms

Restrooms are one of the high-risk areas for COVID-19 transmission! Don't hang out in the restroom any longer than you have to. Use a paper towel to touch faucet and toilet handles and to open doors after you've washed your hands. Don't use air dryers; they can spread virus particles through the air. See Chapter 6: Work! for more tips and tricks on safely using a public restroom.

### Buses and Carpooling

When carpooling or on a bus with others, keep windows down, even if the AC is on. Students who use the bus should sit as far apart from each other as possible, wear masks, and sanitize their hands after getting off the bus. Students or parents/guardians who are carpooling should keep the volume of music or radio low to avoid the need for speaking loudly over the noise. Check that your driver wears a mask and has the right supplies to disinfect seats and doors handles. Bring your driver some bleach wipes or hand sanitizer as a thank you for helping you get to school safely.

## Elementary School Parents/Guardians

Some of the best things you can do for your child are to reassure them, support them, and explain new school and class rules to them. Teach your children proper COVID-19 prevention habits - wearing masks, washing hands, no hugging, and keeping 6 feet away from others. It may be hard for your child to get used to these rules, but it will be easier if you prepare them and reinforce what their teachers recommend.

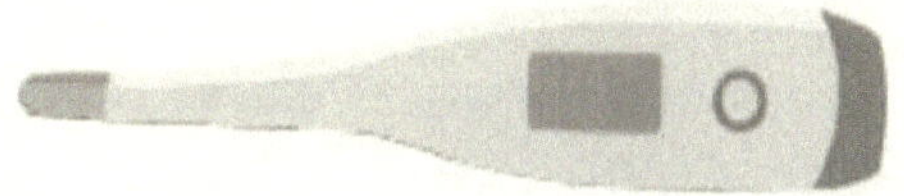

It is important that all students, regardless of age, **stay home if they are sick** - this keeps COVID-19 from getting into schools in the first place!

## Middle and High School Students

Practicing proper COVID-19 prevention habits is especially important for middle and high school students, who interact with more students each day than any other age group. Check your temperature every day before school! (If you are running a fever [oral/skin temperature greater than 100.4°F (38°C)], you should stay home.) Make sure to wear your mask, social distance, and wash your hands frequently. Clean your locker (especially the handle and outside) as you would any other frequently touched surface and wash your hands after using your locker or being in a locker room. See Chapter 6: Work! for more information.

In the cafeteria or food court, choose prepackaged meals or meals served to you by someone using PPE. Avoid buffets and salad bars and do not share drinks or eating utensils with anyone. It's best to bring food from home. **Wash or sanitize your hands for 20 seconds before and after eating** (you may want to keep some lotion with you - your hands will get dry with all that washing!). Stay away from people without masks, especially if they are shouting or talking loudly. Eat outside or in your classroom where you can be far away from others. If you eat in a cafeteria or common area, maintain social distancing.

If your school implements staggered scheduling for arrival, drop-off, or lunch times, be sure you **adhere to the schedules that have been established** - don't go anywhere early or late!

## University Students

As always, proper PPE (especially wearing a mask), hand washing/sanitizing, and social distancing are the best things you can do to keep yourself safe. Check out Chapter 2: Yikes! for more information. **Restrooms, dining areas, and entrances/exits to buildings are the most high-risk areas for COVID-19 transmission.** Pay extra attention to social distancing, disinfecting, and PPE in these areas.

Follow the guidelines set by your university and keep up with communications from administrators.

### Housing

Whether you're living on campus or off campus, there are some ways to ensure you are as safe as possible. When living in residence halls, pay attention to the guidelines set by your school's housing departments. Avoid public spaces, such as kitchens and common areas, and practice social distancing at all times. If there are people in an elevator, wait for another one, or take the stairs and don't touch the hand rails. Exercise is good for you!

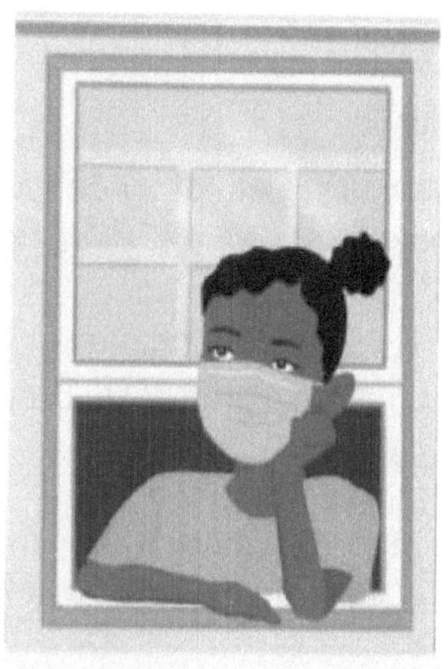

**Open your room's windows** if possible and disinfect frequently touched surfaces (especially doorknobs) often. Consider hanging a shower curtain or other barrier if you and your roommate cannot keep 6 feet apart (for example, if your beds or desks are right next to each other). If you must go to a community bathroom to wash your hands, **keep hand sanitizer in your room** instead. Wear a mask whenever you leave your room.

When using **community bathrooms**, wear a mask whenever feasible. If you must take off your mask to wash your face or brush your teeth, try not to stand directly next to someone. If you can, use the bathroom at times when it is not crowded. See Chapter 6: Work! for more information on how to safely use public restrooms.

**Food**

When using the cafeteria or food court, aim for prepackaged meals or meals served to you by someone using PPE. Avoid buffets and salad bars and do not share drinks or eating utensils with anyone.[84] If available, use disposable plates/cups/eating utensils. If you can, select pre-pay or no-touch payment options. **Wash or sanitize your hands for 20 seconds before and after eating** (you may want to keep some lotion with you, as your hands will get dry with all that washing!). Eat outside or in your room where you can be far away from others. If you eat in a cafeteria or common area, maintain social distancing.

## Prepare Before You Get Sick

If you get COVID-19 while you're away at school, you may have to self-isolate for 10 days without family support. Make a plan with your family at home and your friends at school before you get sick. Make sure you have copies of your insurance card. Go through Chapter 4: Oh No! and stock up on the medication and supplies you will need. Look at Chapter 3: Test! to decide when and how to be tested.

If it's possible, move out of the residence hall/apartment complex until you are better. Otherwise, remain in your room as much as possible. Wear a mask and warn others if you need to leave. Since you live in a crowded high-risk environment, getting tested for COVID-19 is important. If you test positive, people potentially exposed to you (direct contacts, not secondary contacts) will need to be notified and **you must isolate for at least 10 days.** Have a friend drop food off at your door! For much more on how to take care of yourself when sick, see Chapter 4: Oh No! If you test negative but have symptoms, especially fever or cough, please use common sense and assume you have COVID-19. Tests aren't fool-proof - we all need to take care of ourselves and each other!

The question of how to go back to school affects all of us. Authorities everywhere are trying to figure out the best plan. School reentry plans will most likely change as COVID-19 patterns change. For now we can all do our best to keep ourselves safe, avoid the spread of COVID-19, and make sure that students can learn in a safe environment. This means protecting teachers, school staff, families, and students.

We hope that with these guidelines in mind you'll be able to stay healthy at work and at school, but we know that even the best preparation can't guarantee ideal outcomes. In the next chapter, we'll provide some useful tools to help you (or anyone you know) monitor your health and keep track of COVID-19 symptoms, just in case you do get sick.

# Chapter 8

# TRACK! OGT SYMPTOM TRACKER

Use our symptom tracker to match your symptoms with those of COVID-19 and self-monitor changes. Please monitor your symptoms every day for 10 days. Research shows that symptoms can worsen around day 8. Symptoms may appear 2-14 days after exposure. If you seek medical care, bring this symptom tracker with you.

## COVID-19 Symptoms

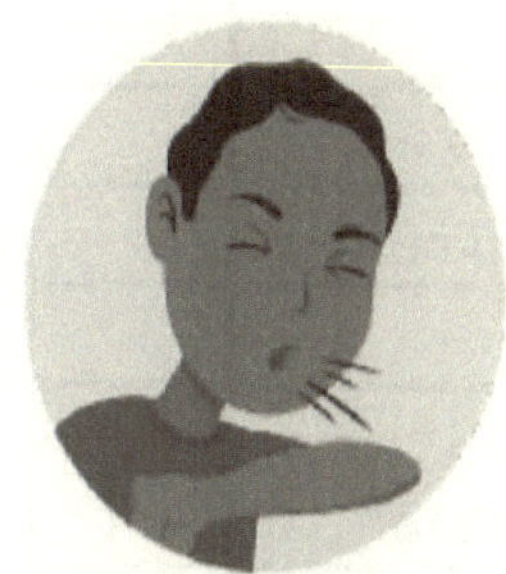

Cough

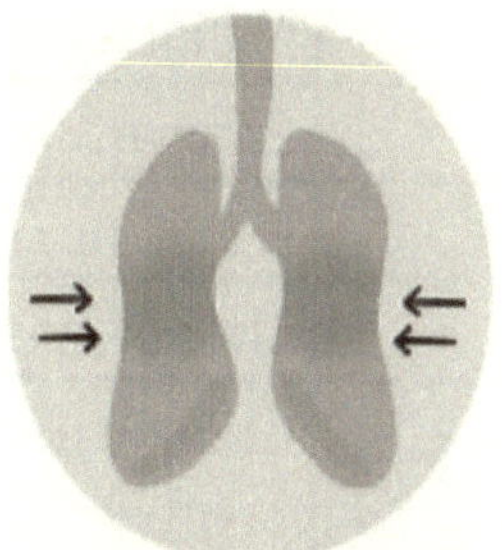

Shortness of Breath

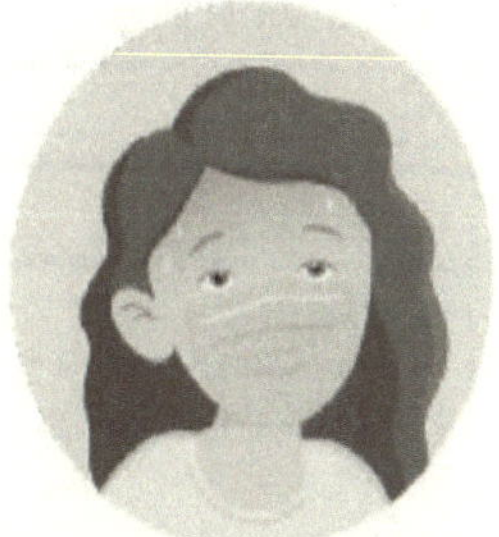

Fever over 100.4 F

If you develop emergency warning signs for COVID-19, get medical attention immediately. Emergency warning signs include*:

* Trouble breathing
* Persistent pain or pressure in the chest
* New confusion or inability to arouse
* Bluish lips or face

*This list is not all inclusive. Please consult your medical provider for any other symptoms that are severe or concerning.[85]

# Charts and Tools

| Full Name | | Current Medical Conditions | |
| --- | --- | --- | --- |
| Age | | | |
| Height | | Current Medication | |
| Weight | | | |
| Date and Time Symptoms Began | | Allergies | |

| Higher Risk Categories (Check all that apply and Provide additional information if necessary) | | | |
| --- | --- | --- | --- |
| Hypertension | | Malignancy | |
| Diabetes | | Postpartum (<6 weeks) | |
| Obesity | | Pregnancy (if yes, trimester) | |
| Asthma | | Liver Disease | |
| Heart Conditions | | Chronic neurological or neuromuscular disease | |
| Lung Conditions | | Immunodeficiency, including HIV | |
| Other(s), please specify | | | |

| Record your symptoms on a scale of 1-5: 1 being normal and 5 being severe. (Print this page twice and record symptoms for 10 days) | | | | | | | | | | |
|---|---|---|---|---|---|---|---|---|---|---|
| Symptom | Day 1 AM | Day 1 PM | Day 2 AM | Day 2 PM | Day 3 AM | Day 3 PM | Day 4 AM | Day 4 PM | Day 5 AM | Day 5 PM |
| Subjective Fever (Y/N) | | | | | | | | | | |
| Cough | | | | | | | | | | |
| Shortness of Breath/ Dyspnea | | | | | | | | | | |
| Fatigue/ Malaise/ Myalgias | | | | | | | | | | |
| Sore throat | | | | | | | | | | |
| Nasal Congestion | | | | | | | | | | |
| Diarrhea/ Nausea/ Vomitting | | | | | | | | | | |
| Other Symptoms | | | | | | | | | | |

| Record the following signs to the best of your ability. (Print this page twice and record signs for 10 days) | | | | | | | | | | |
|---|---|---|---|---|---|---|---|---|---|---|
| Signs | Day 1 AM | Day 1 PM | Day 2 AM | Day 2 PM | Day 3 AM | Day 3 PM | Day 4 AM | Day 4 PM | Day 5 AM | Day 5 PM |
| Fever > 100.4 | | | | | | | | | | |
| Adult O2 Sat % | | | | | | | | | | |
| Child O2 Sat % | | | | | | | | | | |
| Adult Respiratory Rate (breaths per minute) | | | | | | | | | | |
| Child Respiratory Rate (breaths per minute) | | | | | | | | | | |
| Blood Pressure | | | | | | | | | | |

Medicine Tracking Chart: Use this chart to record the date, time, and dose of your medications.

| Date | Time | Medicine | Dose |
| --- | --- | --- | --- |
|  |  |  |  |
|  |  |  |  |
|  |  |  |  |
|  |  |  |  |
|  |  |  |  |
|  |  |  |  |
|  |  |  |  |
|  |  |  |  |
|  |  |  |  |
|  |  |  |  |
|  |  |  |  |
|  |  |  |  |
|  |  |  |  |

# Important Notes

Normal Child Respiratory Rate (Breaths per Minute):

* Less than 2 months: up to 60 breaths per minute
* 2–11 months: up to 50 breaths per minute
* 1–5 years: up to 40 breaths per minute
  * **Tip:** Ask someone else to measure your breaths per minute while you are watching TV or at rest.

Normal Adult Respiratory Rate (Breaths per Minute):

* Normal Adult Respiratory Rate: up to 30 breaths per minute (If you feel short of breath, contact your health provider immediately.)

O2 Saturation:

* Child: O2 Saturation should be over 95%
* Adult: O2 Saturation should be over 95%
  * Use a fingertip oxygen monitor. Take the measurement 2-3 times to get an accurate reading.

If you experience shortness of breath, contact your health provider immediately.

**IF YOU ARE SICK**: Stay home except to get medical care and separate yourself from other people in your home. This is known as home isolation. Wash your hands frequently.

You can stop home isolation if you meet all three of the following conditions:

* You have had no fever for at least 24 hours (one full day) without using medicine to reduce fever

  **and**
* Other symptoms have improved (for example, when your cough or shortness of breath have improved)

  **and**
* At least 10 days have passed since symptoms first appeared.

Always follow your health care provider's recommendations.

# LEGAL DISCLAIMER

*The information contained in the Corona Care Handbook has been sourced from materials published by the following: WHO, CDC, Hesperian Health, Lancet Medical Journal, New England Journal of Medicine, UpToDate, Merck Manual Consumer Version, and PubMed. It is provided for informational purposes only and is not a substitute for the medical advice of your health care provider. Information can change; always check with your healthcare provider and/or CDC.gov.*[86]

# FINAL THOUGHTS

COVID-19 is shaking the foundations of human society. Our families, communities, government, economy, and even our environment are profoundly affected in ways that we are only now beginning to understand.

Strangely enough, during this very public global pandemic, the realization that we are each at risk of COVID-19 creates private and individual questions: What does COVID-19 mean to me personally? How can I take care of myself? Is my family at risk? This is a time of assessing our lives and identifying priorities. The search for guidance as we navigate life with COVID-19 is both personal and universal.

It is our hope that the tools in this handbook will empower you to appropriately manage the risk of illness during this pandemic. **Although this crisis is global, the solution lies in the hands of the individual.** Each of us can safely prevent the spread of this disease. We can educate ourselves, create personal solutions, and take practical, informed steps toward better health.

COVID-19 is a new, worldwide illness, but it's no match for the ingenuity of humanity. We've overcome challenges throughout our development as a civilization. We will continue, together, to grow and to become healthier, more connected members of our shared global community.

Thank you so much for reading our handbook. Use it, share it, print it. **You are now part of the One Good Turn Team, and sharing knowledge is our mission.**

**To Your Health,**

**Ann Messer, MD, Annie Albrecht, and the One Good Turn Team**

P.S. Questions? Comments? Get in touch! **Contact us at**
<u>info@onegoodturn.org</u>

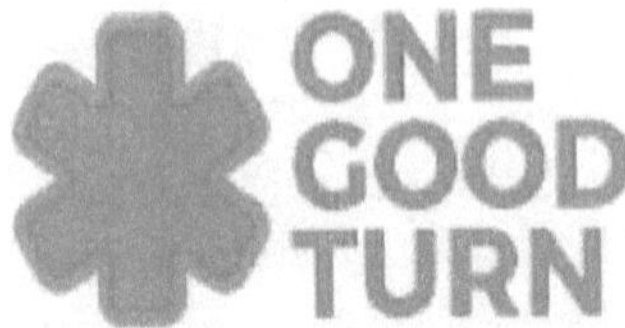

<u>www.onegoodturn.org</u>

# ACKNOWLEDGEMENTS

The Corona Care Handbook is not the work of one author. It is the product of an incredibly hardworking, intelligent, and passionate team. We cannot possibly recognize all of the amazing people who were part of this process here, but we wanted to try.

Thank you, Ann, for your vision and leadership. Thank you for being a dreamer and a doer. Thank you for always reminding us of the importance of our work. Thank you for your determination and dedication to making a difference.

Thank you, Theresa, for your dedication, good natured energy, and medical expertise.

Thank you, Helen, for your creativity and willingness to dive in head first.

Thank you, Addison, for your humor, intelligence, and get-it-done attitude.

Thank you, Ivy, for your attention to detail and astute observations.

Thank you, Mia, for your storytelling abilities and social media magic.

Thank you, Lilian, for your independence, tenacity, and dedication to being one step ahead.

Thank you, Irene, for your persistence, research capabilities, and medical knowledge.

Thank you, Julie, for your incredible copy editing skills, organization, and great questions.

Thank you, Annie, for seeing so long ago what One Good Turn could become and for devoting all of your remarkable and wide-ranging talents toward achieving that goal.

Thank you, Tim, for your patience, understanding, and unwavering support.

Thank you to the amazing folks at Love, Tito's. Your support made this handbook possible. We are honored to work with a foundation that has such a significant and positive impact both locally and globally. Thank you for everything you've done to make the world a healthier and happier place.

And thank you to everyone else who contributed to this remarkable project. We wish we could recognize you all individually but we'd have to add another 100 pages to this book to do so. Instead, please know that we are humbled and so incredibly grateful for your support.

To Your Health,

The One Good Turn Team

# ABOUT THE AUTHORS

## Ann Messer, MD, Founder and Executive Director of One Good Turn

Ann Messer, MD, is a Board Certified Family Physician who has been practicing family medicine and urgent care for 30 years. With over a decade of experience in Global Health, Ann founded One Good Turn to give health workers around the world the tools and knowledge to build self-sustaining, healthy communities. A graduate of Rush Medical School in Chicago, Dr. Messer did her residency work at Harvard in a triad of internal medicine, psychiatry, and family practice. Dr. Messer was named a Fulbright Specialist by the US Department of State for her work developing a clinical competency curriculum in Cambodia. She was recently awarded the Inspire Humanitarian Award by the United Nations Association Austin Chapter. Dr. Messer lives in Austin with her husband Tim; their three grown children are nearby, and together they enjoy outdoor sports, good food, and the family dog, Ziggy.

## About One Good Turn

Ann Messer, MD founded One Good Turn in 2016 after over a decade of work in global health. She learned that despite a lack of access to basic medical education and current health care information, health workers in remote communities are eager to learn and participate in educational opportunities. A humanitarian and a scientist, Ann established One Good Turn to educate, as well as to treat, our global neighbors in neglected communities. Today, our 501(c)(3) partners with local health workers to provide practical medical education and clinical care. Through education, we build sustainable pathways to better health for communities worldwide. Learn more at www.onegoodturn.org

# REFERENCES

**Chapter 1: What is COVID-19?**

1. Bar-On et al., *Science Forum: Sars-CoV-2 (COVID-19) by the numbers*, [
   2020
2. Holdeman, *COVID-19: Transmission Scenarios Explained*, May 11, 202
3. CDC, *Older Adults*, June 25, 2020
4. Abbas, *The Mutual Effects of COVID-19 and Obesity*, May 6, 2020
5. Zhu et al., *Association of asthma and its genetic predisposition with th
   severe COVID-19*, n.d.
6. The Lancet, *Viral dynamics in mild and severe cases of COVID-19*, Mar
   2020
7. Heneghan et al., *SARS-CoV-2 viral load and the severity of COVID-19*, [
   2020
8. Yu et al., *Quantitative Detection and Viral Load Analysis of SARS-CoV-
   Infected Patients*, July 28, 2020
9. WHO, Transmission of SARS-CoV-2: implications for infection prever
   precautions, July 9, 2020

**Chapter 2: Yikes COVID-19 is Everywhere**

10. MacIntyre & Chughtai, *A rapid systematic review of the efficacy of fac
    and respirators against coronaviruses and other respiratory transmissi
    viruses for the community, healthcare workers and sick patients*, April
    2020
11. East Alabama Medical Center, *Why Wearing a Mask is Important*, n.d
12. WHO, *Advice on the use of masks in the context of COVID-19*, June 5, 2
13. CDC, *Strategies for Optimizing the Supply of Facemasks*, June 28, 202
14. CDC, *People with Disabilities*, July 24, 2020
15. CDC, *Considerations for Wearing a Mask*, July 16, 2020

16. Hill, *From the Frontlines: The Truth About Masks and COVID-19*, June ...
17. Vanderbilt University Medical Center, *Coronavirus (COVID-19) Inforn for Employees and Patients*, July 6, 2020
18. CDC, *How to Wear Masks*, July 6, 2020
19. Streeter, *20-second Disney songs to wash your hands to*, n.d.
20. CDC, *Handwashing: Clean Hands Save Lives*, n.d.
21. FDA, *FDA Updates on Hand Sanitizers with Methanol*, n.d.
22. Lindberg, *How to Make Your Own Hand Sanitizer*, July 6, 2020
23. U.S. Department of Homeland Security, *S&T's Research, Developmen Testing and Evaluation (RDT&E) Efforts re COVID-19*, April 13, 2020
24. Anfinrud et al., *Visualizing Speech-Generated Oral Fluid Droplets with Light Scattering*, May 21, 2020
25. Hamner et al., *High SARS-CoV-2 Attack Rate Following Exposure at a ( Practice — Skagit County, Washington, March 2020*, May 12, 2020
26. CDC, *Cleaning Your Home*, May 27, 2020
27. EPA, *List N: Disinfectants for Use Against SARS-CoV-2 (COVID-19)*, July 2020
28. Gargiulo, *Fact check: It's true, Clorox Splash-Less bleach does not disin surfaces*, June 15, 2020
29. Clorox, *Clorox Splashless Bleach*, n.d.
30. FDA, *Fraudulent Coronavirus Disease 2019 Products*, n.d.
31. CDC, *Cleaning Your Home*, May 27, 2020
32. FDA, *Shopping for Food During the COVID-19 Pandemic - Information Consumers*, May 1, 2020
33. CDC, *Characteristics of Adult Outpatients and Inpatients with COVID-i 3, 2020
34. CDC, *How to Quit Smoking*, n.d.
35. Hesperian Health Guides, *COVID-19: Breathing*, n.d.
36. American Lung Association, *Breathing Exercises*, May 27, 2020
37. Bentley, n.d.
38. Emanuel et al., *COVID-19 Risk Index*, June 30, 2020


## Chapter 3: TEST! All about Testing, Your Results, and Exposure risks


39. Texas Medical Association, *Been Exposed to COVID-19?*, July 23, 2020

40. CDC, *Test for Current Infection*, July 23, 2020
41. CDC, *Test for Past Infection*, June 30, 2020
42. FDA, *Coronavirus Testing Basics*, July 2020
43. CDC, *State and Territorial Health Department Websites*, n.d.
44. NACCHO, *Directory of Local Health Departments*, n.d.

## Chapter 4: OH NO! I have COVID-19!

45. Streeter, *20-second Disney songs to wash your hands to*, n.d.
46. McIntosh, *Coronavirus disease 2019 (COVID-19): Clinical features*, July 2020
47. National Institutes of Health, *Vitamin C*, n.d.
48. Hesperian Health Guides, *COVID-19: Breathing*, n.d.
49. American Lung Association, *Breathing Exercises*, May 27, 2020
50. CDC, *Ending Home Isolation*, July 20, 2020

## Chapter 5: HELP! I'm Taking Care of Someone with COVID-19

51. National Institutes of Health, *Potent antibodies found in people recov from COVID-19*, June 30, 2020.
52. CDC, *Cleaning Your Home*, May 27, 2020
53. EPA, *List N: Disinfectants for Use Against SARS-CoV-2 (COVID-19)*, July 2020
54. CDC, *Frequently Asked Questions*, August 4, 2020
55. Han et al., *Viral RNA Load in Mildly Symptomatic and Asymptomatic C with COVID-19, Seoul*, October 2020
56. CDC, *Multisystem Inflammatory Disease in Children*, n.d.
57. CDC, *Ending Home Isolation*, July 20, 2020

## Chapter 6: WORK! How am I going to handle this?

58. CDC, *Telebriefing Update on COVID-19*, June 25, 2020
59. Dockery et al., *The Ocular Manifestations and Transmission of COVID- Recommendations for Prevention*, May 8, 2020
60. Kehres, *UNC Chemistry Scholar Shows You How to Make a DIY Emerge*

Face Shield_, April 8, 2020
61. CDC, _When and How to Wash Your Hands_, n.d.
62. CDC, _Detailed Disinfection Guidance_, July 10, 2020
63. CDC, _How to Make Strong (0.5%) Chlorine Solution from Liquid Bleach_
64. EPA, _List N: Disinfectants for Use Against SARS-CoV-2 (COVID-19)_, July 2020
65. CDC, _Worker Safety and Support_, July 28, 2020
66. OSHA, _Guidance on Preparing Workplaces for COVID-19_, n.d.
67. CDC, _What to Do if You're Sick_, May 8, 2020
68. CDC, _Ending Home Isolation_, July 20, 2020
69. U.S. Department of Labor, _Families First Coronavirus Response Act: Er Paid Leave Rights_, n.d.
70. CDC, _Businesses & Workplaces_, August 4, 2020
71. CDC, _Handwashing in Community Settings_, n.d.
72. EPA, _List N: Disinfectants for Use Against SARS-CoV-2 (COVID-19)_, July 2020
73. FDA, _Food Code_, 2017
74. CDC, _Worker Safety and Support_, July 28, 2020

## Chapter 7: SCHOOL! How do I Learn Safely?

75. CDC, _People with Disabilities_, April 7, 2020
76. Johns Hopkins University, _eSchool+ Initiative Analysis of School Reop Plans_, n.d.
77. CDC, _Operating Schools_, May 19, 2020
78. Raman, _How to Safely Get Vitamin D From Sunlight_, April 28, 2018
79. CDC, _Detailed Disinfection Guidance_, July 10, 2020
80. CDC, _Cleaning and Disinfection for Community Facilities_, May 27, 202
81. Jang et al., _Cluster of Coronavirus Disease Associated with Fitness Dan Classes, South Korea_, August 2020
82. Vanderbilt University Medical Center, _Coronavirus (COVID-19) Inform for Employees and Patients_, July 6, 2020
83. Hamner et al., _High SARS-CoV-2 Attack Rate Following Exposure at a ( Practice — Skagit County, Washington, March 2020_, May 12, 2020
84. Johns Hopkins University, _Johns Hopkins University eSchool+ Initiativ

_Analysis of School Reopening Plans_, n.d.
85. Johnson, _Black light experiment shows how quickly a virus like Covid-_
    _spread at a restaurant_, May 14, 2020

## Chapter 8: TRACK! OGT Symptom Tracker

86. CDC, _Symptoms_, May 13, 2020

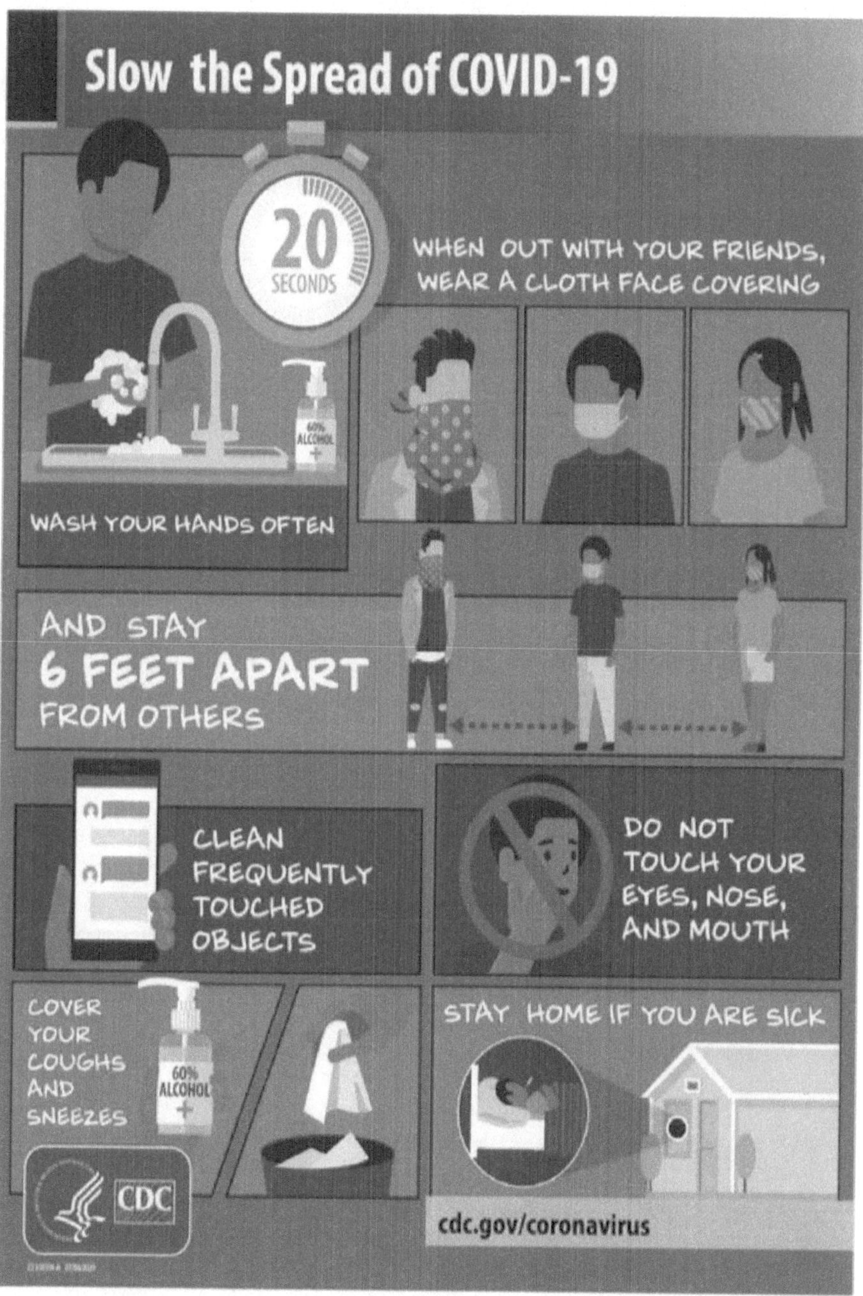

Slow the Spread of COVID-19
20 SECONDS
60% ALCOHOL
WASH YOUR HANDS OFTEN
WHEN OUT WITH YOUR FRIENDS, WEAR A CLOTH FACE COVERING
AND STAY 6 FEET APART FROM OTHERS
CLEAN FREQUENTLY TOUCHED OBJECTS
DO NOT TOUCH YOUR EYES, NOSE, AND MOUTH
COVER YOUR COUGHS AND SNEEZES
60% ALCOHOL
STAY HOME IF YOU ARE SICK
CDC
cdc.gov/coronavirus

# 10 things you can do to manage your COVID-19 symptoms at home

Accessible Version: https://www.cdc.gov/coronavirus/2019-ncov/if-you-are-sick/steps-when-sick.html

**If you have possible or confirmed COVID-19:**

1. **Stay home** from work and school. And stay away from other public places. If you must go out, avoid using any kind of public transportation, ridesharing, or taxis.

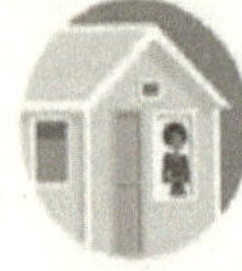

2. **Monitor your symptoms** carefully. If your symptoms get worse, call your healthcare provider immediately.

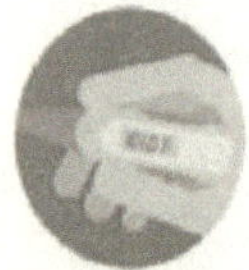

3. **Get rest and stay hydrated.**

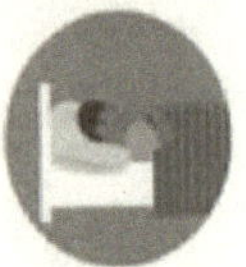

4. If you have a medical appointment, **call the healthcare provider** ahead of time and tell them that you have or may have COVID-19.

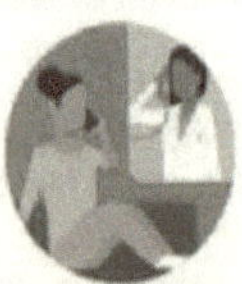

5. For medical emergencies, call 911 and **notify the dispatch personnel** that you have or may have COVID-19.

6. **Cover your cough and sneezes.**

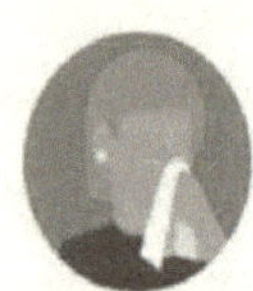

7. **Wash your hands often** with soap and water for at least 20 seconds or clean your hands with an alcohol-based hand sanitizer that contains at least 60% alcohol.

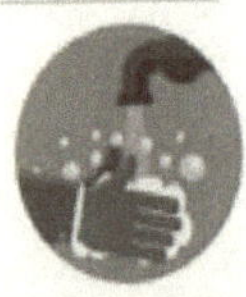

8. As much as possible, stay in a specific room and **away from other people** in your home. Also, you should use a separate bathroom, if available. If you need to be around other people in or outside of the home, wear a cloth face covering.

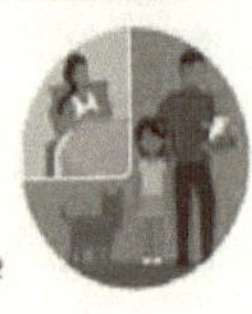

9. **Avoid sharing personal items** with other people in your household, like dishes, towels, and bedding.

10. **Clean all surfaces** that are touched often, like counters, tabletops, and doorknobs. Use household cleaning sprays or wipes according to the label instructions.

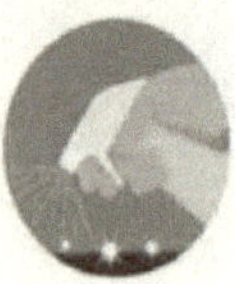

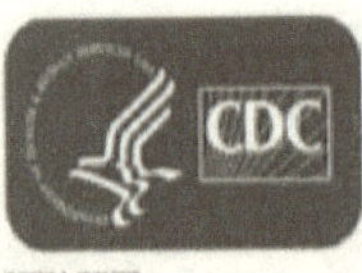

cdc.gov/coronavirus

# COVID-19
CORONAVIRUS DISEASE

## BE INFORMED:

### Know Your Risk During COVID-19

*On a scale of 1 to 10, how risky is...*

Ranked by physicians from the TMA COVID-19 Task Force and the TMA Committee on Infectious Diseases.

Please assume that participants in these activities are following currently recommended safety protocols when possible.

TEXAS MEDICAL ASSOCIATION
Physicians Caring for Texans

|  |  |  |
|---|---|---|
| 1 | Opening the mail | LOW RISK |
| 2 | Getting restaurant takeout | |
| 2 | Pumping gasoline | |
| 2 | Playing tennis | |
| 2 | Going camping | |
| 3 | Grocery shopping | LOW-MODERATE |
| 3 | Going for a walk, run, or bike ride with others | |
| 3 | Playing golf | |
| 4 | Staying at a hotel for two nights | |
| 4 | Sitting in a doctor's waiting room | |
| 4 | Going to a library or museum | |
| 4 | Eating in a restaurant (outside) | |
| 4 | Walking in a busy downtown | |
| 4 | Spending an hour at a playground | |
| 5 | Having dinner at someone else's house | MODERATE RISK |
| 5 | Attending a backyard barbecue | |
| 5 | Going to a beach | |
| 5 | Shopping at a mall | |
| 6 | Sending kids to school, camp, or day care | |
| 6 | Working a week in an office building | |
| 6 | Swimming in a public pool | |
| 6 | Visiting an elderly relative or friend in their home | |
| 7 | Going to a hair salon or barbershop | MODERATE-HIGH |
| 7 | Eating in a restaurant (inside) | |
| 7 | Attending a wedding or funeral | |
| 7 | Traveling by plane | |
| 7 | Playing basketball | |
| 7 | Playing football | |
| 7 | Hugging or shaking hands when greeting a friend | |
| 8 | Eating at a buffet | HIGH RISK |
| 8 | Working out at a gym | |
| 8 | Going to an amusement park | |
| 8 | Going to a movie theater | |
| 9 | Attending a large music concert | |
| 9 | Going to a sports stadium | |
| 9 | Attending a religious service with 500+ worshipers | |
| 9 | Going to a bar | |

**Texas Medical Association** | 401 W. 15th St. | Austin, TX 78701-1680

www.texmed.org | @texmed | @wearetma

Source

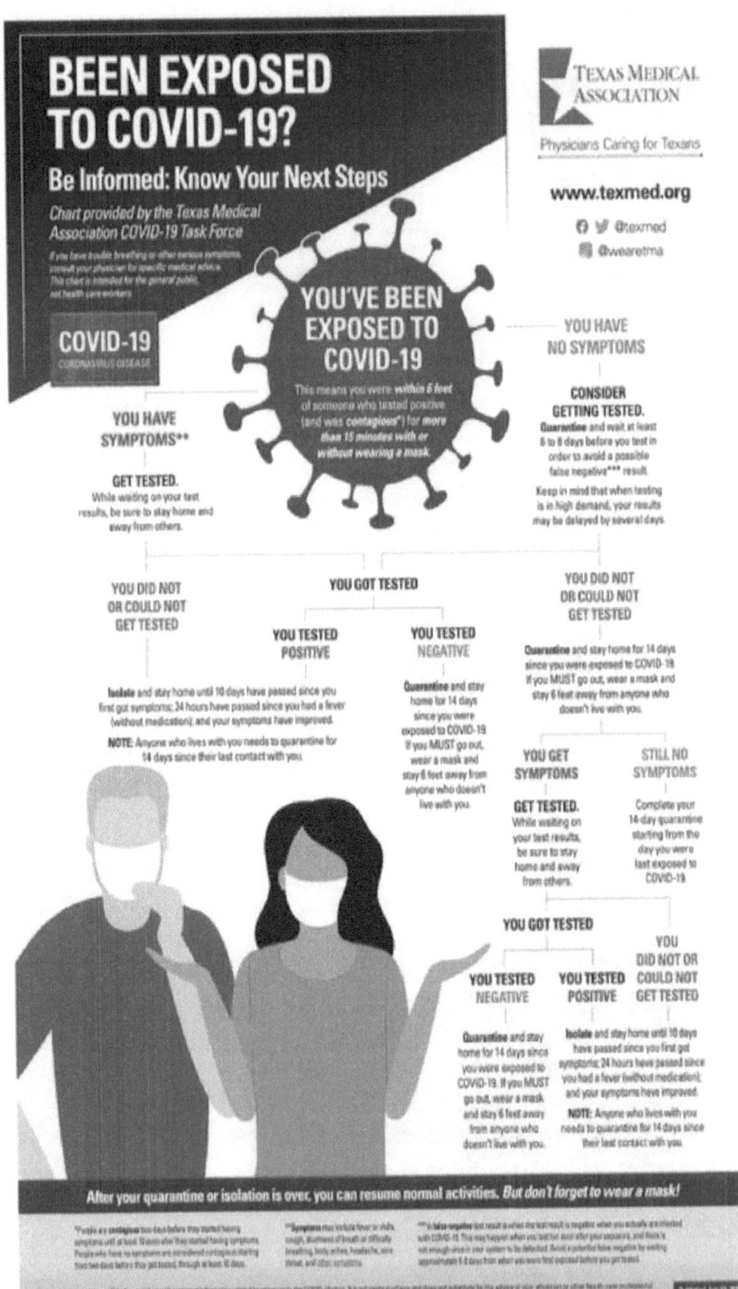

BEEN EXPOSED TO COVID-19?
Be Informed: Know Your Next Steps
Chart provided by the Texas Medical Association COVID-19 Task Force
If you have trouble breathing or other serious symptoms, consult your physician for specific medical advice. This chart is intended for the general public, not health care workers.
COVID-19
CORONAVIRUS DISEASE
TEXAS MEDICAL ASSOCIATION
Physicians Caring for Texans
www.texmed.org
@texmed
@wearetma
YOU'VE BEEN EXPOSED TO COVID-19
This means you were within 6 feet of someone who tested positive (and was contagious*) for more than 15 minutes with or without wearing a mask.
YOU HAVE SYMPTOMS**
GET TESTED.
While waiting on your test results, be sure to stay home and away from others.
YOU HAVE NO SYMPTOMS
CONSIDER GETTING TESTED.
Quarantine and wait at least 5 to 8 days before you test in order to avoid a possible false negative*** result.
Keep in mind that when testing is in high demand, your results may be delayed by several days.
YOU DID NOT OR COULD NOT GET TESTED
YOU GOT TESTED
YOU TESTED POSITIVE
YOU TESTED NEGATIVE
YOU DID NOT OR COULD NOT GET TESTED
Isolate and stay home until 10 days have passed since you first got symptoms; 24 hours have passed since you had a fever (without medication); and your symptoms have improved.
NOTE: Anyone who lives with you needs to quarantine for 14 days since their last contact with you.
Quarantine and stay home for 14 days since you were exposed to COVID-19. If you MUST go out, wear a mask and stay 6 feet away from anyone who doesn't live with you.
Quarantine and stay home for 14 days since you were exposed to COVID-19. If you MUST go out, wear a mask and stay 6 feet away from anyone who doesn't live with you.
YOU GET SYMPTOMS
GET TESTED.
While waiting on your test results, be sure to stay home and away from others.
STILL NO SYMPTOMS
Complete your 14-day quarantine starting from the day you were last exposed to COVID-19
YOU GOT TESTED
YOU TESTED NEGATIVE
YOU TESTED POSITIVE
YOU DID NOT OR COULD NOT GET TESTED
Quarantine and stay home for 14 days since you were exposed to COVID-19. If you MUST go out, wear a mask and stay 6 feet away from anyone who doesn't live with you.
Isolate and stay home until 10 days have passed since you first got symptoms; 24 hours have passed since you had a fever (without medication); and your symptoms have improved.
NOTE: Anyone who lives with you needs to quarantine for 14 days since their last contact with you.
After your quarantine or isolation is over, you can resume normal activities. But don't forget to wear a mask!
Published June 12, 2020

[1] Bar-on et al., *SARS-CoV-2 (COVID-19) by the numbers*, 2020

[2] CDC, *Duration of Isolation and Precautions for Adults*, July 22, 2020

[3] CDC, *When to Quarantine*, August 3, 2020

[4] CDC, *How it Spreads*, June 16, 2020

[5] MacIntyre & Chughtai, *A rapid systematic review of the efficacy of face masks and respirators against coronaviruses and other respiratory transmissible viruses for the community, healthcare workers and sick patients*, April 30, 2020

[6] East Alabama Medical Center, *Why Wearing a Mask is Important*, n.d.

[7] WHO, *Advice on the use of masks in the context of COVID-19*, June 5, 2020

[8] CDC, *Strategies for Optimizing the Supply of Facemasks*, June 28, 2020

[9] CDC, *People with Disabilities*, July 24, 2020

[10] The Clear Mask, *Clear Mask*, n.d.

[11] CDC, *Considerations for Wearing a Mask*, July 16, 2020

[12] Hill, *From the Frontlines: The Truth About Masks and COVID-19*, June 18, 2020

[13] Vanderbilt University Medical Center, *Coronavirus (COVID-19) Information for Employees and Patients*, July 6, 2020

[14] CDC, *How to Wear Masks*, July 6, 2020

[15] Streeter, *20-second Disney songs to wash your hands to*, n.d.

[16] CDC, *Handwashing: Clean Hands Save Lives*, n.d.

[17] Off The Beaten Path Bookstore

[18] FDA, *FDA Updates on Hand Sanitizers with Methanol*, n.d.

[19] Lindberg, *How to Make Your Own Hand Sanitizer*, July 6, 2020

[20] U.S. Department of Homeland Security, *S&T's Research, Development, Testing and Evaluation (RDT&E) Efforts re COVID-19*, April 13, 2020

[21] Anfinrud et al., *Visualizing Speech-Generated Oral Fluid Droplets with Laser Light Scattering*, May 21, 2020

[22] Hamner et al., *High SARS-CoV-2 Attack Rate Following Exposure at a Choir Practice — Skagit County, Washington*, March 2020, May 12, 2020

[23] CDC, *Cleaning Your Home*, May 27, 2020

[24] EPA, *List N: Disinfectants for Use Against SARS-CoV-2 (COVID-19)*, July 30, 2020

[25] Gargiulo, *Fact check: It's true, Clorox Splash-Less bleach does not disinfect surfaces*, June 15, 2020

[26] Clorox, *Clorox Splashless Bleach*, n.d.

[27] FDA, *Fraudulent Coronavirus Disease 2019 Products*, n.d.

[28] CDC, *Cleaning Your Home*, May 27, 2020

[29] FDA, *Shopping for Food During the COVID-19 Pandemic - Information for Consumers*, May 1, 2020

[30] CDC, *Characteristics of Adult Outpatients and Inpatients with COVID-19*, July 3, 2020

[31] CDC, *Telebriefing Update on COVID-19*, June 25, 2020

32  CDC, *How to Quit Smoking*, n.d.

33  CDC, *Pregnancy Data*, August 6, 2020

34  CDC, *Pregnancy and Breastfeeding*, June 25, 2020

35  The Clear Mask, *Clear Mask*, n.d.

36  **National Institutes of Health, Vitamin C, n.d**

37  Hesperian Health Guides, *COVID-19: Breathing*, n.d.

38  American Lung Association, *Breathing Exercises*, May 27, 2020

39  Emanuel et al., *COVID-19 Risk Index*, June 30, 2020

40  CDC, *State and Territorial Health Department Websites*, n.d.

41  NAACHO, *Directory of Local Health Departments*, n.d.

42  US Department of Health and Human Services, *Community Based Testing Sites for COVID-19*, n.d.

43  CDC, *Test for Current Infection*, July 23, 2020

44  CDC, *Symptoms*, May 13, 2020

45  Streeter, *20-second Disney songs to wash your hands to*, n.d.

46  McIntosh, *Coronavirus disease 2019 (COVID-19): Clinical features*, July 15, 2020

47  National Institutes of Health, *Vitamin C*, n.d.

48  Hesperian Health Guides, *COVID-19: Breathing*, n.d.

49  American Lung Association, *Breathing Exercises*, May 27, 2020

50  CDC, *Ending Home Isolation*, July 20, 2020

51  National Institutes of Health, *Potent antibodies found in people recovered from COVID-19*, June 30, 2020.

52  CDC, *Cleaning Your Home*, May 27, 2020

53  EPA, *List N: Disinfectants for Use Against SARS-CoV-2 (COVID-19)*, July 30, 2020

54  National Institutes of Health, *Vitamin C*, n.d.

55  CDC, *Frequently Asked Questions*, August 4, 2020

56  Han et al., *Viral RNA Load in Mildly Symptomatic and Asymptomatic Children with COVID-19, Seoul*, October 2020

57  CDC, *Multisystem Inflammatory Disease in Children*, n.d.

58  CDC, *Ending Home Isolation*, July 20, 2020

59  CDC, *Telebriefing Update on COVID-19*, June 25, 2020

60  Dockery et al., *The Ocular Manifestations and Transmission of COVID-19: Recommendations for Prevention*, May 8, 2020

61  Kehres, *UNC Chemistry Scholar Shows You How to Make a DIY Emergency Face Shield*, April 8, 2020

62  CDC, *When and How to Wash Your Hands*, n.d.

63  CDC, *Detailed Disinfection Guidance*, July 10, 2020

64  EPA, *List N: Disinfectants for Use Against SARS-CoV-2 (COVID-19)*, July 30, 2020

65  CDC, *Worker Safety and Support*, July 28, 2020

66  OSHA, *Guidance on Preparing Workplaces for COVID-19*, n.d.

67  CDC, *What to Do if You're Sick*, May 8, 2020

68  CDC, *Ending Home Isolation*, July 20, 2020

69  U.S. Department of Labor, *Families First Coronavirus Response Act: Employee Paid Leave Rights*, n.d.

70  CDC, *Businesses & Workplaces*, August 4, 2020

71  CDC, *Handwashing in Community Settings*, n.d.

72  EPA, *List N: Disinfectants for Use Against SARS-CoV-2 (COVID-19)*, July 30, 2020

73  FDA, *Food Code*, 2017

74  CDC, *People with Disabilities*, April 7, 2020

75  Johns Hopkins University, *eSchool+ Initiative Analysis of School Reopening Plans*, n.d.

76  CDC, *Operating Schools*, May 19, 2020

77  Raman, *How to Safely Get Vitamin D From Sunlight*, April 28, 2018

78  CDC, *Detailed Disinfection Guidance*, July 10, 2020

79  CDC, *Cleaning and Disinfection for Community Facilities*, May 27, 2020

80  Jang et al., *Cluster of Coronavirus Disease Associated with Fitness Dance Classes, South Korea*, August 2020

81  Vanderbilt University Medical Center, *Coronavirus (COVID-19) Information for Employees and Patients*, July 6, 2020

82  Hamner et al., *High SARS-CoV-2 Attack Rate Following Exposure at a Choir Practice — Skagit County, Washington, March 2020*, May 12, 2020

83  Johns Hopkins University, *eSchool+ Initiative Analysis of School Reopening Plans*, n.d.

84  Johnson, *Black light experiment shows how quickly a virus like Covid-19 can spread at a restaurant*, May 14, 2020

85  CDC, *Symptoms*, May 13, 2020

86  CDC, *Use of Agency Materials*, n.d.

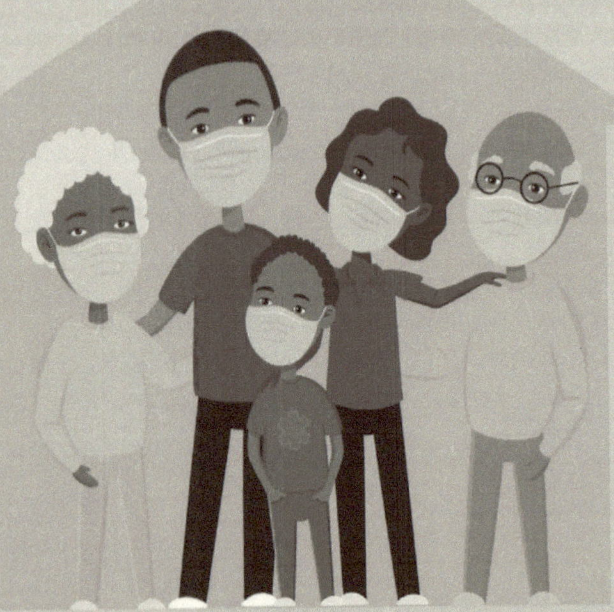

STAY SAFE!
WWW.ONEGOODTURN.ORG
ONE GOOD TURN